The Weight Loss Coach

Simple Solutions To Lasting Weight Loss

Benjamin Bonetti

I've dedicated this book to my wife and children who have supported me through both my personal and professional growth.

CONTENTS

Acknowledgments   9

Introduction   11

Chapter One   15

How This Book Works For You   15
Excuses   16
Why Do We Eat?   18
What Is Digestion?   19
What Is Insulin?   21
What Is Glycogen?   23
What Are Food Groups?   25
What Are Carbohydrates?   26
What Are Proteins?   29
What Are Fats?   31
Stimulants   35

Chapter Two   39

What Is The Metabolic Rate?   39
Why Is RMR Important?   40
Measuring RMR   41
The Problem With the Way We Think   43

Chapter Three   47

Benefits Beyond Weight Loss   47
A Few Points to Get Started   48
Motivation   51
Skinny-Fat and Fat-Fat, DON'T Be Fooled   53
Why Do You Want to Lose Weight – Please Be Honest!   55
What You Should Be Doing   58

BOOTCAMP WORKOUT # 1   59
BOOTCAMP WORKOUT # 2   60

Chapter Four   **63**

Nutrition – You Are What You Eat   63
Do You Need Organic/Raw?   63
Frozen Vs Fresh   65
Preparing the Feast – Eye Candy?   66
Is Fresh the Solution?   68
Getting Back to the Basics of Living …   70
Kitchen Basics   72
The First Step   73
Get Local   74
Stop Talking About It and Start Doing It   75

Chapter Five   **81**

Food – More Than Just Food   81
The Foods You Eat Vs. The Lifestyle You Live   84
Reality Check   85
Tomorrow is a better day …   89
What Do You Value?   90
Remember the Art of Replacement   92
Isn't It Time You Started Listening to Your Body?   93
You Only Live Twice   95
Time Vs. Benefits With Food Production   96
Challenges – How Are You Going to Get Over Them?   97

Chapter Six   **101**

5 Healthy Breakfasts   102
5 Healthy Lunches   105
10 Healthy Dinners   108

Mindful Tasks   **119**
Exercises   **125**
About Benjamin   **135**

ACKNOWLEDGMENTS

I remember when I was first introduced to the world of fitness some 20 years ago I was overwhelmed with the mass of conflicting advice and I looked at the leaders, hoping that I one day would have their knowledge and skill. But, one thing I have since learned is that the industry, both then and now, is still preaching very much the same thing – nothing original or cutting edge as they would like you to believe.

Cutting Out The Ball (That's Me)

I'm not about re-packaging old content, I'm about building functional fitness strategies that work for the masses and do not require expensive equipment or specialist nutritional ingredients; I'm about using what you already have access to and what's within reach for most.

I know that if you have to add more to your already busy life, then it's unlikely that you'll able to commit, not because you don't want to but because you just can't.

It's because of this that I acknowledge not the working professionals within the fitness industry or the highly qualified and skilled nutritionists, but every person who spends the time and commits to making a programme work for them. That's you.

It's you that I'm grateful for; the feedback you provide inspires me to reach out and help all those willing to listen. I acknowledge those who listen, commit and perform – thank you and good luck.

INTRODUCTION

When I started out in my career I didn't know how much of an impact I would have on those I worked with, I was just excited about what I was able to offer through my passion for learning and my motivation to improve the life of those around me – through coaching, fitness and nutrition.

I'm a realist and despite being aware of the many different quick fix solutions out there, this is not an approach you will encounter with me – I say it how it is. If you've signed up to my way of thinking then you're in it for the long-haul. This is a code of practice I set in place for myself at the very beginning and refused to change despite on-going pressure to sell the 'quick fix' solution that many insisted I try – not naming any well-known weight loss shakes preached by Multi-Level-Marketing schemes.

I've been very fortunate along my path to work with some amazing people, including friends and family whom I've often bored with my constant excitement about the topic and my inner desire to improve the lives of those around me, yet they ultimately benefited – whether they liked it or not.

I'm serious about nutrition, fitness and lifestyle performance…

During sessions many years ago, it dawned on me that there was a serious issue with 'health and fitness' education here in the UK. Nutritional advice was hard to come by and I came to the realisation that the masses of conflicting fitness advice created a minefield for anyone genuinely trying to find a simple solution. It was because of this that my goal shifted from just providing set exercises to looking at the whole picture. I gave up working with those with one goal – to lose weight quickly – and focused on working with those who wanted to improve their life for the better and for the long-term. I studied psychology and many other mental therapies as well as trained in alternative medicine.

Quickest way to lose weight? Don't put it on in the first place.

Taking this all-rounded approach to fitness, and not signing up to 'one' set belief, separated me from the majority of 'fit-pros' and I'm glad. I'm glad because my clients have one of the highest success rates in the country and benefit from not only getting fit but meeting a new path of life that offers an abundance of lifestyle changes.

It's expected that nearly 80% of the UK will be obese within the next 15 years. Why? Well, I'll cover all of the aspects within this book, hopefully removing you from this statistic in the process.

When were you taught to be healthy?

....

....

What type of lifestyle are you sold on a daily basis?

....

....

Nothing in life is guaranteed but what you do today controls your life in the future and therefore influences what you are likely to become. You have the choice right now whether to improve or not. The action you take today directly influences your life tomorrow – it really is as simple as that.

Taking the right action today will change the way you live your life moving forward; you can either carry on living your life the way you are now and staying as you are now or you can take action today to change. Ultimately, the choice is yours to make.

We humans are the problem – we accept what is being sold to us without questioning it.

I believe this book will change the way you think about your life and your ability to achieve, and it will hopefully inspire you to move forward with a healthier and more fulfilling life.

Best wishes

Benjamin x

CHAPTER ONE

How This Book Works For You

Within this book I will be questioning some of the things you may believe to be true and for this reason there may be some points that confuse you or perhaps don't make sense when compared to things you've been taught. However, I ask that you trust me, despite what you may think I know what I'm talking about.

We'll be looking at functional fitness. This is a term I use a lot and it represents something that's really important to me and the message I deliver. For example, if you are currently 23 stone, then I'm not going to ask you to train for a marathon in 12 weeks, likewise, if you are underweight and want to gain muscle, I'm not going to recommend fasting. Functional fitness is all about providing each individual with the information needed to achieve their individual goals through a combination of education, accountability and practical advice that will work within their life. We're all different and it would be unfair of me to ask everyone to follow the same programme. Only *you* can decide what *you* want to achieve.

I will be covering simple science but this isn't anything you should be worried about as I'll be sticking to the basics and going into just enough depth to keep you interested. We'll go through a lot of information quickly with the emphasis being on grasping the relevance of what is being said rather than delving into deeper scientific issues. Of course, you can always choose to do further research on areas that particularly interest you.

Here are some questions to help kick-start your thinking:

If you know that it's bad to eat processed foods that are high in fat, why do you do it?

....

....

What is your motivation to lose weight and improve your health?

....

....

Excuses

Let's be honest from the very beginning – you're busy. I know this. I also know you've tried lots of diets before – and you've been told they're the best! You want results but deep down you know that committing to something that doesn't interest you isn't going to work – despite knowing it's something you *should* be doing. This is a common issue, and it's the reason why you have perhaps yo-yo dieted in the past.

I'm not going to patronise you with endless facts about the scientific structure of the molecule, nor am I going to tell you that you need to achieve a six-pack in order to be normal. What I will do is provide you with workable strategies that have helped my clients achieve the lasting results they want. There isn't a set programme for you to follow but instead, a set of ideas designed to help you get from where you are now to where you want to be.

Why are you unhappy with the weight you are?

....

....

What have you done to really change in the past?

....

....

Why do your diets usually fail?

....

....

I want you to stop right now: stop reading: stop what you're thinking about, and just read over the answers you've given above. Immerse yourself in each question and really think about the reasons *why...*

Why is now the right time to change?

....

....

Why can't I allow this to continue anymore?

....

....

What do I need to do to ensure I change for good?

....

....

"Definiteness of purpose is the starting point of all achievement."
–W. Clement Stone

Why Do We Eat?

In the most simplistic terms we eat because we need to – at a
deeper level, and in a more natural sense, our craving is survival
(taste is a craving that has evolved over time). The primary role
and purpose of food is the production of energy. The foods we
eat are processed by our digestive system to extract the energy
which is then distributed to the rest of our body to enable us to
function. Obviously, it's a little more complicated than that but
we don't need to go into the intricacies of biochemistry for the
purposes of this book. However, it's a really interesting subject and
I would recommend taking the time to read more about it when you
advance.

The digestion process can be broken down into five broad stages:

1. We consume food via the mouth. This is chewed and
    swallowed to begin its journey through to the stomach and
    so on.

2. Glucose is extracted from the consumed food (highlighting
    the importance of consuming quality food).

3. Glucose is passed around the body via the bloodstream by

demand.

4. Energy is extracted and used.

5. Any unused energy is stored as fat (highlighting the importance of regulating the amount consumed).

In brief, you can see how over indulgence, lack of movement and fat retention are linked. This is something we'll explore in more detail later. For now, the important message to take on board is that the amount you consume, the amount used, and the amount stored all start out as the choice you make to introduce the food into your system.

Notice the language here, 'you', 'your'...

Throughout the book you will notice the language I use indicates that *you* have to take ownership over your diet. Reading the book is a great start but it's the actions you take as a result of reading it that will create the impact you desire.

What Is Digestion?

Digestion can be described simply as the process of breaking food down to a point at which the body can absorb the nutrients contained within it. The process begins in the mouth with teeth helping to break the food down into smaller pieces. Saliva also plays an important role at this stage as it contains enzymes which work to further break down the fats and carbohydrates.

When the food becomes broken down enough to be swallowed, it passes through the throat into the stomach. This is where the real magic happens: the food is further broken down by a number of liquids produced by the stomach, each one with its own role to play. The makeup of the food determines the speed at which it will be broken down but as a basic guide, carbohydrates are processed faster than protein and protein faster than fat.

As the food leaves the stomach, it's pretty much in a refined liquid form. It passes into the gastrointestinal tract where most of the absorption happens. There are many different levels of absorption but for the moment we're going to focus only on the absorption of glucose.

Glucose is absorbed through the cell walls and used to make energy. In the same way that you refuel your car according to the distance you've travelled and the distance you've yet to travel, your body needs to be refuelled according to its energy needs. If you don't refuel it often enough, you're going to break down, but if you overfill it in one refuelling, it's going to spill over. Of course, this is an overly simplistic breakdown of the whole process but providing in depth information on the role of mitochondria and membranes at this stage would only lead to you feeling overwhelmed and more likely to switch off. I'm choosing to keep it simple because I want you to stay switched on to the idea of following through with the recommendations I make.

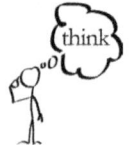

Why is it important that I consume the right amount of food for my energy output (distance travelled)?

....

....

Could this be a reason why I've gained weight in the past?

....

....

What changes can I make to ensure that when I move more I consume more, and consume less when I move less?

....

....

What Is Insulin?

When I mention insulin, most people think about diabetes. Insulin is a complex subject covering a wide variety of factors but, in a nutshell, insulin is needed to enable glucose to enter the body's cells to make energy. However, in modern western cultures there is now an issue arising over having too much glucose in the body as the excess is stored as fat. Insulin can also cause an increase in appetite, and this can of course be a major issue for those looking to control or lose weight – especially if they don't manage the production of insulin consciously.

So why is insulin important? Well, insulin grabs excess glucose in the blood and stores it as glycogen in the liver and muscles. This naturally leads to a drop in the insulin levels in the blood which in turn causes a signal to be sent to the brain to trigger an increase in appetite and the need to eat. When the amount of insulin in the body is matched by the body's energy requirements, things run smoothly, but issues kick-in when there's an imbalance. Consuming a daily diet of sugary fast foods can create an imbalance known as insulin resistance which is now a major cause of obesity and cardiovascular illnesses in the modern world.

Eating a quality diet free of highly processed and refined foods can massively change the way insulin is produced and used by the body. Insulin can be thought of as a tin miner in the body, breaking down the sugars and passing them on to be used immediately as fuel or storing them away for later use. The more sugar there is for the tin miner to deal with, the more there is to be stored away when it's not needed, and all of this leads to an untidy workplace on a cellular level.

Quality in and quality out; rubbish in and rubbish out.

So what's the solution? When you think about it, removing ALL processed foods and foods that are high in sugar from your diet is the simplest and most straightforward way to help the tin miner get his workplace in order. Replacing those foods with fresh, non-processed foods containing only natural sugars and minerals gives the body the energy supplies it needs without the clutter of excess making the tin miner's job harder than it needs to be.

What foods do I consume that are high in refined (or white) sugars?

....

....

Would now be a good time to remove them from my diet?

....

....

What naturally grown foods (that I like) could I replace them with?

....

....

When can I implement this change in my diet?

....

....

Important note: when removing processed and 'fake' foods from your diet, you're going to experience a number of shifts within the body. Just as a drug addict goes through a withdrawal, you'll experience a similar effect with the impact generally leading to symptoms such as diarrhoea, headaches, mood swings, stomach cramps and emotional ups and downs. This isn't anything to be concerned about and the symptoms usually ease after only a couple of days. Keep in mind that any negative effects you experience are only temporary and they are simply the by-product of your body craving and detoxing at the same time.

What Is Glycogen?

As glucose levels build up within the blood, insulin takes on a second role. The glucose that can't be absorbed through the cell walls is converted into glycogen which is essentially the short-term fuel source used by the body in everyday activities. Only limited amounts of glycogen are stored by the body as it's in constant use which means that stored sugars (fat) are called upon when fuel supplies are low. The more active we are and the more we deplete glycogen supplies, the more we use stored sugar (glucose) supplies, thus controlling the build-up of fat held within the body.

It's the additional fitness activities we take part in that are usually most relevant here. As we increase the energy requirement of the body, the more likely it is that we'll begin dipping into the body's fat reserves to fuel the additional activity. However, it can take newcomers to exercise a little while to begin reaping the rewards of 'fat burning' in this way as it takes repeated additional energy demands to effectively shock the body into letting go of reserves.

Increasing our activity levels or simply moving more changes the dynamics of energy production and this, along with a change in diet from fake sugars to natural sugars, brings with it MASSIVE results.

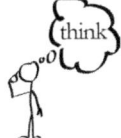

Why is fitness important to the fat burning process?

. . . .

. . . .

What can I do to increase the movement within my normal working day?

. . . .

. . . .

What adjustments should I make to ensure that my body doesn't store additional sugars?

. . . .

. . . .

In Summary

The process is as follows:

> Food is consumed - glucose is produced - circulates within the blood - enters the cells - used as fuel (energy).

Keeping optimum levels of glucose in your blood is essential in your weight loss journey. The more aware you become and the more knowledgeable you are in terms of how your body functions, the more likely it is that you will be able to consciously control your food choices and ultimately reduce your sugar (fat) intake.

It's quite possible that the above information is all stuff you already knew but there's a big difference between *knowing* about something and *doing* something about it, right? The only thing that's important now is that you make a conscious decision to change; you must *choose* to make changes for the better and you must *commit* to following through on your choice. The more leverage you create in this choice, the less likely you are to relapse into old habits along the way.

What Are Food Groups?

Something I'm regularly asked to explain is the difference between one type of food and another. This is often because people struggle to create a healthy balance in their daily diet and it's something we'll look at in more detail later but for now, try asking yourself the question below. Very often, the answer to this one question is all you need to help you figure out whether you're making a good food choice.

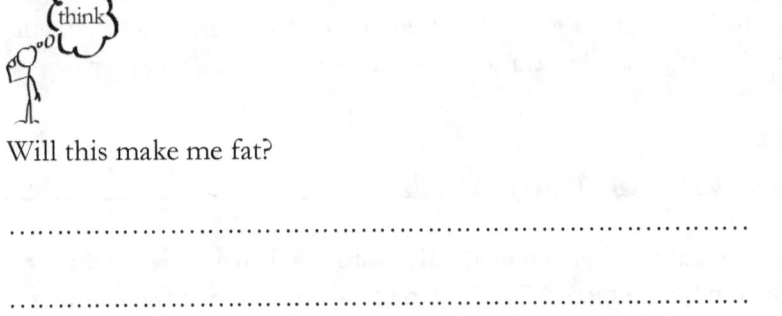

Will this make me fat?

....

....

Now, I appreciate the harshness of this question but the reality is that you need to start looking at your food with a completely different set of eyes – and you need to start asking better questions. For example, if a pizza has rocket and pineapple on it, does that make it a healthy choice; do 'light' versions of cheese or butter make a food the right choice? The answer is no.

We often over complicate food but making good choices needn't be hard. In fact, understanding food choices is the easiest aspect of weight loss but, that being said, there are three food groups you need to be aware of to help you make better choices – carbohydrates, proteins and fats. Each food group acts differently and has a different role within the body, and ultimately each group is broken down at a different speed thus providing the body with the right things at the right times.

In order (based on most foods):

> Carbohydrates are usually the first to be broken down as they provide the 'instant' energy needed for everyday functioning.

> Proteins are usually the second to be broken down and they are used to build and repair all areas of the body.

> Fats are the last to broken down and they are used as insulation and energy reserves.

Now let's look at these in a little more detail, but again it's my intention to keep things simple and relevant. My recommendations are just that, recommendations, and it must always be remembered that the best diet for you is one that will last forever; a diet that will keep you motivated to eat well and make better choices every day.

What Are Carbohydrates?

Carbohydrates are generally divided into two categories and are the main source of glucose. They are made from groups of sugars that are linked in varying lengths and as a result perform differently depending on the lifestyle you lead and environmental factors. Carbohydrates are usually sourced from widely grown crops and offer a more affordable food choice compared to fats and proteins.

1. Simple Carbohydrates

Simple carbohydrates are a sub-group typically made up of short chains and usually digested faster than longer chain complex carbohydrates. The speed of digestion and absorption into the body is measured by an index known as the Glycaemic Index (or GI) and simple carbohydrates sit at the high end of the scale indicating a rapid release of energy.

Simple carbohydrates are more commonly found in western diets where processed and refined foods are more available and as such are a large contributing factor to weight gain and retention.

Examples include:

All desserts (other than whole fruit), ice cream, sherbet, frozen yogurt, most breads, many crackers (100% stoneground whole grain crackers are okay), cookies, cakes, muffins, pancakes, waffles, pies, candy, chocolate (dark, milk and white), breaded or battered foods, all types of dough (filo, pie crust), most cereals, most pastas, noodles and couscous, jellies, jams and preserves, bagels, pretzels, pizza, potato chips, peanut butter containing sweeteners, puddings and custards, crisps, granola bars, power bars, energy bars, most rice and corn cakes, fried vegetable snacks, ketchup, sweetened yogurts and other sweetened dairy products, honey-roasted nuts, fizzy drinks.

Looking at the above, what stands out?

....

....

How many of the above do you have on a daily basis?

....

....

What could you do to remove simple carbohydrates from your diet?

....

....

Complex Carbohydrates

Complex carbohydrates are made from longer chains of sugars and take longer to be digested by the body. They also contain more fibre than simple carbohydrates and the slower release of energy places them at the lower end of the Glycaemic Index (GI).

Examples include:

Fresh/frozen meat, poultry, seafood, fresh or frozen unsweetened fruits, all vegetables (other than white potatoes), parsnips, beets, carrots, whole grains (whole grain rice, oats, barley, quinoa, corn), nuts and seeds of all types, unsweetened nut butters, unsweetened coconut, popcorn, 100% whole grain rice cakes, whole legumes (beans, peas, lentils), guacamole, unsweetened salsa, olives, unsweetened pickles, eggs, soy products (like tofu and soy milk), unsweetened all-natural dairy products (milk, plain yogurt, cheeses, butter), 100% stoneground whole grain breads or crackers without added sugar, unsweetened coffee, tea, sparkling water (either plain or with natural flavours or essences added), water, unsweetened tomato sauce and other unsweetened, starch-free sauces, unsweetened salad dressings, herbs and spices, oils, unsweetened vinegars (balsamic vinegar and certain other fruity vinegars can be very sweet so check labels for carbohydrate content), textured vegetable protein, tempeh.

Looking at the above, what stands out?

....

....

How many of the above do you have on a daily basis?

....

....

What action could you take today to introduce more complex carbohydrates into your life?

....

....

Which Carbohydrate Is Better?

Hopefully, you will have noticed from the examples above that there is one clear distinction between simple and complex carbohydrates. Simple carbohydrates are most likely to be found in manufactured and highly processed foods whereas complex carbohydrates are most likely to be found in foods that have remained close to their natural state (i.e. the way they were grown).

This makes complex carbohydrates the better choice for those looking to control insulin levels (slower energy release prevents insulin spikes) or anyone embarking on a weight loss journey. Both types have a purpose and it's unlikely that you will go completely without one or the other but the slower release of energy provided by complex carbohydrates helps to keep hunger at bay by creating a satisfying feeling of being 'full' for longer.

TASK

Make it a conscious decision to choose ingredients that have remained close to their natural state and you won't go far wrong. When creating your shopping list, refer back to the complex carbohydrates mentioned above and try to replace processed simple carbohydrates with more natural complex carbohydrate options.

What Are Proteins?

Proteins are extremely complex and in reality there are only a few relevant things you need to know at this stage. Firstly, proteins are made up of amino acids which are the building blocks for all of the body's tissue. Your physiological proteins consist of 20 different amino acids and although your body requires all of them, you only have the ability to synthesize some of them. The remainder, those your body can't manufacture, must be sourced from the foods in your diet or you run the risk of developing a protein deficiency.

Current recommendations state that to meet your body's protein needs, you must consume a minimum of 0.8 grams of high quality protein per each kilogram of your bodyweight (or 0.4 grams per pound) per day. This is considered adequate in terms of meeting your essential amino acid requirements and it's an interesting fact, but really there is no need for the majority of people to consciously manage their protein intake in this way.

Secondly, protein is found mainly in animal products so meat is the primary source unless you are vegetarian. Glucose can also be found in protein sources but due to the longer breakdown period required, carbohydrates remain the body's main source of energy.

Examples of High Quality Protein Foods:

Soya beans, cheese, venison, pumpkin seeds, crunchy peanut butter, skinless chicken breast, sunflower seeds, skinless turkey breast, boneless salmon fillets, sardines, almonds, beef fillet, lamb steak, pork chops, crab meat, cod, shrimp, haddock, bacon, couscous, anchovies, pork sausages, eggs, goji berries, cottage cheese, tofu, porridge oats, hummus, brown rice, peas, yogurt, broccoli, coconut, whole milk, asparagus, spinach.

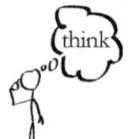

Looking at the above list, what immediately stands out to you?

....

....

How many of the high protein foods listed do you consume on a daily basis?

....

....

How do you currently get sufficient protein?

....

....

Your protein, as far as we are concerned, should come from natural (notice the trend on words) ingredients. So, although a chicken dipper contains a chicken of sorts, it shouldn't be considered a suitable source of high quality protein. The same applies to the following:

Corned beef, prosciutto, salami, supermarket bacon, bologna, hot dogs, mortadella, turkey dinosaurs etc.

What Are Fats?

Firstly, let's bust the myth that fats are bad. Sure, some fats are bad and most modern 'known' fats come into this category, but there are also good fats and it's essential that we get enough of them in our diet as a diet too low in fat can lead to skin problems, inhibit the body's control of inflammation and adversely affect blood pressure. Basically, there are two groups of fats you need to know about:

1. Saturated fats
These are the bad fats associated with heart disease and known to be detrimental to overall health. Common sources are meat

fat, butter, cheese, and processed foods such as cakes and biscuits.

2. Unsaturated fats

These can be split into two further groups:

Monounsaturated fats – these are the good fats known to be of benefit to overall health. Common sources are oils such as olive, groundnut and rapeseed, and they're also found in seeds and nuts.

Polyunsaturated fats – these also have positive health benefits in that they can help to lower unhealthy blood cholesterol levels. Polyunsaturated fats are also important in that they contain essential fatty acids which the body can't produce by itself. However, it's now known that they may also reduce *healthy* levels of blood cholesterol so a combination of polyunsaturated and monounsaturated fats is needed in the diet to achieve a healthy balance. Common sources are vegetable fats and oily fish.

The Bad Fats

The fats to eat sparingly or to avoid altogether in your diet are saturated fats and trans fatty acids. Both are linked with raised cholesterol levels, clogged arteries, and an increased risk of developing heart disease.

Saturated fats are found in animal products and the common sources mentioned above, also eggs and vegetable fats that are liquid at room temperature, coconut and palm oils for example. It's recommended that saturated fats should make up no more than 10% of your total daily calories, and ideally less than 5%.

The Good Fats

Both mono and polyunsaturated fats, when eaten in moderation, can help to lower cholesterol levels and reduce your risk of developing heart disease.

Monounsaturated fats form a large part of the diet in Mediterranean countries, olive oil in particular, and this is thought to be the reason for low levels of heart disease in these areas. Typically liquid at room temperature but solid when refrigerated, these heart-healthy fats are a good source of vitamin E, a health-boosting antioxidant which is often lacking in our diets, and can be found in olives, avocados, hazelnuts, almonds, Brazil nuts, cashews, sesame seeds, pumpkin seeds, and olive, canola, and peanut oils.

Much heralded omega-3 fatty acids are one type of polyunsaturated fat, found in fatty fish (salmon, trout, catfish, mackerel), as well as flaxseed and walnuts. Oily fish contains the 'long-chain' type of omega-3s which are known to be particularly effective in terms of lowering the potential to develop heart disease.

TASK

Remove all cooking oils made from animal fats and all vegetable or 'fake' fats from your kitchen.

There is evidence to back up claims that saturated fats can increase the risk of developing colon and prostate cancers so we recommend, whenever possible, choosing healthy unsaturated fats and consciously striving to achieve and maintain a healthy weight.

We also hear a great deal about trans fatty acids or trans fats these days but it's important to be aware that there are two types: the naturally occurring type found in small amounts in dairy and meat, and the artificial type found in liquid oils that are hardened/ processed into 'partially hydrogenated' fats. The naturally occurring types are not of particular concern, especially if you choose low-fat dairy products and lean meats, but the artificial types should be avoided. They're used extensively in frying and found in baked goods, cookies, icings, crackers, packaged snack foods, microwave popcorn, and some varieties of margarine.

Examples of Good Fats:

Olive oil, canola oil, peanut oil, sesame oil, avocados, olives, nuts (almonds, peanuts, macadamia nuts, hazelnuts, pecans, cashews), peanut butter, soybean oil, corn oil, safflower oil, walnuts, sunflower, sesame, and pumpkin seeds, flaxseed, fatty fish (salmon, tuna, mackerel, herring, trout, sardines), soymilk, tofu.

What is apparent to you having looked at the good fats listed above?

....

....

What bad fats do you have at home?

....

....

Why would now be a good time to throw them away?

....

....

It's unlikely that you will be able to remove all 'bad' fats from your diet completely but you should still be consciously aware of what you're eating at all times. Pay attention to what's in the foods you eat at home as well as when you're eating out or grabbing a bite on the go. Take note, fats are very good at being hidden.

> WARNING: avoid the temptation to buy anything with 'light', 'reduced fat', 'low calorie', 'low fat' or anything else suggesting a food represents a healthier option. Anything with a FAT WARNING on the label probably wasn't good enough to eat in the first place.

Stimulants

For me, stimulants are anything you consume to cause a rapid change in the natural production and release of chemicals within the body – a sugar rush, a caffeine boost, a legal high if you like. These sorts of stimulants have become commonplace over recent years with a well-known 'energy drink' and a plethora of coffee shop chains leading the trend. As I see it, socially accepted stimulants are just as bad as the not so social and illegal varieties, yet they don't get the same bad press. However, the fact remains that in effect they are *all* potentially damaging to health, and here's why…

The long-term effects are still unknown; especially with unnatural stimulants which increase the chemical content within the body.

The mid-term effects are known to be health related issues and illnesses, not forgetting they are addictive.

The short-term effects are a change in the way the body functions.

The most common socially accepted stimulants are as follows:

Sugar: If your goal is to lose weight and remain healthy then you need to take note of this. You will have to remove 'fake' sugars from over 80% of your diet. Now, I'd like to say remove *all* fake sugar but this is highly unrealistic and hard to manage unless you have the time and you feel really serious about adopting a RAW style diet (ideal but sometimes not practical).

Salt: Like fats, there are different types of salts to be considered; there are the good and the bad. The good are those found in plants and the sea – these contain healthy minerals and offer the same taste value as the bad salts. For example, Himalayan Pink Salt is a pure, hand-mined salt that's derived from ancient sea salt deposits and is believed to be the purest form of salt available. The salt crystals range in colour from white to varying shades of pink and deep reds, the result of a high mineral and iron content. The bad salts are the processed varieties, therefore most table salts Table salt is typically mined from underground salt deposits and heavily processed to eliminate minerals, with most varieties containing an additive to prevent clumping. Salt causes a mixed message to be sent to the brain as it's dehydrating but also sends signals of hunger.

Caffeine: I love my coffee, so I'm writing this with great care to avoid sounding hypocritical. Caffeine is *the* high drink and it has become one of the most readily accepted means of socialising on a daily basis. We all know the 'caffeine kick' effect but what most fail to realise is that over consumption is counterproductive. The effects are short-lived and actually inhibit the release of naturally occurring chemicals, meaning the end result is similar to the highs and lows of sugar spikes and crashes. Of course the coffee alone is not the only issue. Added extras such as sugar, syrup and milk all add to the daily consumption of fats – most of which go unnoticed or are forgotten about.

Alcohol: Again, I also enjoy the occasional glass of wine but as far as the body is concerned, alcohol is a sugar, thereby a stimulant and inhibitor. Alcohol reduces the body's ability to absorb minerals and nutrients, it plays with the body's thermostat, and it also causes insulin spikes, thereby generating fat storage. This means that as far as weight loss is concerned it simply doesn't help, actually reducing the speed at which fat is digested and removed from the body.

Tobacco: Nothing positive can be said about the consumption of tobacco. The effects on the body are horrific and the effect it has on weight loss and gain are dramatic. If you smoke, now is the time to stop. However, it's important to avoid the temptation to opt for some form of substitute that will replicate the effects. If you stop and you feel the need to hold something, opt for a carrot. If you need a break out of the office, make a fruit tea, and if you need a replacement, opt for a healthy juice. Patches and all other forms of fake cigarette are still bad for your health, despite the positive packaging and marketing. I used to smoke – so I know.

TASK

1. Remove 'fake' salts from your diet and throw away all table salts from your cupboards. Replace them with natural organic varieties, but still use sparingly. These can be ordered online or picked up from local health food stores, but always check to make sure they don't have any additives included.

2. Over the coming weeks, reduce any caffeine consumption to the minimum. For example, one coffee per day and not after 6pm. It will take seven days to re-set, restore and kick-start the natural production on inhibited chemicals in your body. Avoid the temptation to reach for energy drinks and allow your body to regain control.

3. If you have no intention of cutting out alcohol completely, then reduce your consumption to about six units per week, aiming to then cut to five, then to four units.

4. Stop smoking: go cold turkey. If you need to, book into a spa for a long weekend or stop prior to enjoying a 7-day juice detox. The lengthening of life, not to mention the financial saving, should be enough for anyone to seriously act right now.

CHAPTER TWO

What Is The Metabolic Rate?

Our metabolic rate is the rate at which our body burns calories.
Many people understand the metabolic rate to be a major factor
in determining how quickly or how easily they can lose weight,
but along with this understanding comes the potential for a great
deal of misunderstanding as people find themselves confused
with conflicting advice and theories. It's because of this that I
recommend you take your time over the next section to ensure you
fully digest and understand what is being said. If you need to, fold
over this page and refer back to it over the coming days.

Gaining this knowledge is a very important element of getting
things right in terms of maintaining a healthy body and being able
to control your weight. However, you might be tempted to flick
past it so it's my intention to give you just enough information to be
of benefit without giving you too much and switching you off as a
consequence.

It Is Important...

THE BASICS – Our body burns calories for the energy necessary
to maintain the vital involuntary activities such as breathing,
maintenance of heat, heartbeat and blood circulation, and the
activities of the nervous system and internal organs. Once we go
beyond these functions we burn a lot more calories in everyday
activities such as walking, climbing stairs, working out, playing
sport, even just carrying the shopping.

Our metabolism has a direct bearing on the amount of energy used in each activity so a baseline is needed in order to measure how efficiently our body is burning calories overall to provide us with this energy. To do this we refer back to the amount of energy we use to support our systems when the body is at rest. This baseline measurement can be taken on two levels and they are known as our BMR or RMR.

I will be referring to RMR but be aware that BMR is similar. It's not my intention to throw abbreviations around, I find it annoying when other people do so, but bear with me as all will become clear.

- **BMR** stands for Basal Metabolic Rate and is synonymous with Basal Energy Expenditure or BEE. True BMR measurements are typically taken in a darkened room with the subject resting in a reclining position having just woken up after eight hours of sleep and 12 hours of fasting to ensure the digestive system is inactive.

- **RMR** stands for Resting Metabolic Rate and is synonymous with Resting Energy Expenditure or REE. An RMR measurement is typically taken under less restricted conditions compared to a BMR measurement and the subject doesn't need to spend the night sleeping in a test facility to create the optimum environment for testing.

Why Is RMR Important?

RMR is important because it's a measure of the minimum number of calories we burn in a day – effectively the amount of fuel we need to just keep our engine ticking over at idle. If we know how many calories we burn and we have knowledge of how many calories we consume (eat), then we have a useful tool to work with when we are looking at changing our weight.

It is logical that if we are burning more calories than we are eating then something has to happen. Just what happens is perhaps more complicated than it looks so let's begin with the basic concept of RMR.

For each pound or kilo of body weight we carry we need energy to sustain it. Muscle requires slightly more energy to maintain than fat which is why it becomes easier to lose fat as we gain more muscle. Our vital organs require a LOT more energy than our muscles but overall it averages out.

Measuring RMR

We can estimate our RMR with a formula called the Mifflin-St Jeor equation. It looks like this:

$$H= (99.0\text{-weight}) + (6.25\text{-height}) - (4.92\text{-age}) + 166\text{-sex} \ (1 \text{ for males}; 0 \text{ for females}) - 161$$

If maths is not your thing it probably looks quite daunting but it's a useful gauge in terms of telling us what our expected RMR is based on our height, weight and age. The immediate conclusion many people reach is that if they can reduce their calories to say 1000 calories a day, then the equation is out of balance. They would be burning 2000 calories and eating only 1000, and as the body needs to make up the difference, they would lose weight.

The first little fact we need to consider here is not the main deal, but it's interesting. Most dieticians seem to agree that one pound of fat is about equivalent to 3500 calories of stored energy – that's about 7500 calories per kilo. If you can reduce your calorie intake to 1000 less than your RMR you will potentially lose 1000 calories of body fat a day, or about two pounds/one kilo a week.

The trouble with this is that in most cases, and from my vast knowledge of dealing with people in real life and not from a textbook, your body is just too efficient and it simply slows down your metabolic rate to meet the level of calorie intake. This means that in most cases dieting slows your metabolism which leads to having less personal energy, lower concentration levels, and everything becoming a chore as you just don't feel good.

On the other hand, a high metabolic rate or 'fast' metabolism leads to feeling that you have energy to do everything. This can of course make a huge difference to the way you live your life. Our current lifestyle of fast foods and convenience foods can fool us into believing we are eating lots but there is very little nutrition getting down to the cells of our body so it believes we are starving and consequently slows our metabolic rate right down.

If we are going to reverse this, we need to ensure that our body is getting all the nutrition it needs at a cellular level. Once we've done this, we can drop the calorie intake and our metabolic rate will stay high. However, we have further problems in that the food available to us on supermarket shelves is grown in nutrient deficient soils, picked green so it ships well, stored for too long, and if it's pre-packaged it's normally over-processed. There just isn't enough nutrition in our food to sustain us, and if we look at botanical factors and the active ingredients in our food with things like the amino acids then we are in real trouble.

For the energy equation to be transferred into weight change i.e. the food we eat less the energy we burn equalling net gain or net loss in daily energy, we need to provide our body with all the nutrition it needs on a daily basis so that it doesn't fight against starvation by slowing down our metabolic rate. Something else to realise is that weight gained through a slower metabolism is most likely going to be stored on hips, thighs and stomach.

In summary, if someone has told you that a diet means removing calories, they are wrong. What they should be saying is that it means improving the *quality* of the calories you consume. **Slowing down your metabolic rate does not and will not support a healthy lifestyle.**

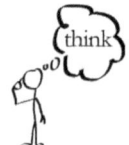

What is my RMR using the calculation below?

....

....

H= (99.0-weight) + (6.25-height) - (4.92-age) + 166-sex (1 for males; 0 for females) - 161

Is my diet providing me with enough energy to perform?

....

....

What adjustments could I make to improve my body's functioning through food?

....

....

The Problem With The Way We Think

If you have tried dieting in the past and it hasn't worked for you, then it's likely that the deeper rooted issues were not addressed. Sure, cutting calories and exercising or trying the latest fad pill may have had some effect, but the chances are the weight sprung back on in no time at all, right?

If this is you, then it's nothing to be ashamed of. You are like the many other millions of people around the world looking for a solution to a problem that they have identified, and for that alone you should congratulate yourself and be happy. Identification is the first step, knowledge the second, and action the third.

Reading this book is already improving your knowledge so let's look ahead to the mind and the thinking behind the actions stage.

"We not only become like those we mix with, but like those we think about the most."

The above is something I say a lot, and for one very good reason. What we think about becomes the way we communicate with ourselves internally and, as a result, is then projected in our behaviours.

Think fat and that's what you'll become...

FACT: more people start a diet for aesthetic reasons rather than lifestyle choices, and their actions are usually driven by a celebrity or a large organisation promoting the idea for one reason only – to make money.

Although there is a degree of financial motivation involved in the writing this book, my main aim is to share the knowledge I have so that I may help you to improve your life and make changes for the better. Sure, money helps, but my main objective is to help you get results. It's for this reason that I ask one thing of you – question the motives behind those glossy adverts that show you rapid weight loss results in return for investing in a certain product, and at the same time, question why obesity is an on-going and growing concern.

These 'mind-plays' have caused many misconceptions about food and they generalise people who adopt a certain way of living.

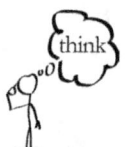

Think for a moment about what comes to mind when you read the following:

Hippy

Bodybuilder

Vegan

Piscetarian

Now think about how you perceive their environments – a hippy based environment, a bodybuilder's environment, vegan, and Piscetarian – what images are created in your mind; how do you see those people living, and what do their environments look like? Now think about the last time you saw an old picture of yourself and remember the way the image made you feel. Were you repulsed, upset, angry, lost for words?

What pictures did you create about yourself?

....

....

What didn't you like about those internal images?

....

....

Why is now the right time to change that perception forever?

....

....

What happens if you don't make the changes needed?

....

....

What we see internally generally manifests into external behaviour and creates a perception we act upon. Now let's pause for a moment and think long term. Think ahead to a moment in the future when you have achieved your ideal weight and imagine looking back at an image of yourself as you are now.

What would you say to yourself?

. . . .

. . . .

I ask you to do this because weight loss or dietary adjustments should be looked at as long term projects, and with a slightly different objective to others you may have had in the past.

CHAPTER THREE

Benefits Beyond Weight Loss

Approaching weight loss or diet with the sole goal of losing weight is never productive, nor is it healthy. Changing your approach to focus on the three areas of nutrition, fitness and lifestyle will bring mental, emotional and physical benefits that complement your whole life, not just the way you look. I've found that those who keep the weight off are those who choose to follow my overall lifestyle changes.

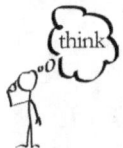

How much better would your life be if you were the weight you wanted to be and you didn't have to think about it ever again?

....

....

Aiming to be a healthy weight is different to aiming for weight loss. Being healthy incorporates every aspect of your future life, not just your body image, and eliminates many other negative aspects of a poor diet such as bloating, skin conditions, lack of energy and low levels of concentration. The choice you make right now depends on the answers you give to these two questions:

1. Do you actually want to lose weight?
2. Why do you want to lose weight?

The answers to these questions generally indicate the 'value' factor involved in the overall process, or the mindful aspect of it all. It's also being able to give honest answers to these questions that will release you from the emotional shackles holding you back.

To start change you must first be open to change.

A Few Points To Get Started

Accept that you *can* be happy right now. With many things, there's often the temptation to wait until the timing is right or the universe is perfectly aligned to give you want you want before making a start. Sadly, and again having worked with many different people, the right time will usually end up being no time. When you start to shift from the 'then' to the 'now' you begin to free yourself up from past problems and future potential issues.

It's only by living in the moment that you can start to take action on the person you are right now and thus change the path you're likely to follow. Avoid the temptation to wait until some future date to make these changes to your life – take charge right now… now… now…

Why do I deserve to be happy and have everything I want in life?

....

....

Why haven't I done what I really wanted so far in my life?

....

....

Look at the reason *why*. To start with, you're not the only person with issues or bad past experiences or anything else negative so GET OVER IT. This may seem harsh but the reality is that the longer you live in the past, the longer you will be tormented with whatever negativity it had to offer. The root cause of weight gain for most people is a traumatic event that spiralled into comfort frenzy... and the rest is history.

Now, don't get me wrong, I know that things can be tough but how about choosing to deal with things differently. When times get tough, or you're hurt, or something negative happens, how about reaching for something positive that will assist you rather than reaching for the cookie jar? Just imagine for a moment what it would be like to reach out and ask for help (no shame in asking for help when you need it) rather than folding in and adding to the bad news by reaching for the cookie jar; what would happen if you actively chose to do something that would support you in a healthy and long-term positive way?

Why have I been holding on to past negative issues?

....

....

What comfort have they provided?

....

....

When would be the right time to let go?

....

. . . .

Why haven't I let go in the past?

. . . .

. . . .

What will happen if I don't let go right now?

. . . .

. . . .

Next, you need to commit to being the person you want to be. We all have choices in life; to have or to have not, to stand alone and allow others to follow, or to become lost in the crowd and be forgotten. With weight loss, as with any other kind of change, you have to commit to making change happen. Without commitment, making changes in the areas of your life that need attention becomes impossible and you will never achieve the full life you want or the memories that go with it.

"The most difficult thing is the decision to act, the rest is merely tenacity." – **Amelia Earhart**

For me, commitment basically means to follow through on what you said you would do. Being able to commit also says a lot about the strength of a person. The irony is that it takes the same degree of commitment to live a healthy lifestyle and be healthy as it does to choose *not* to live a healthy lifestyle and be unhealthy. Ultimately, the more enjoyment you get out of doing something, the more you're encouraged to do it again but if it's a chore then that's the emotional connect you will have with anything that resists you along your path.

Why am I *now* committed to making the necessary changes in my life?

....

....

What will my life look like 20 years from now if I continue living the way I do?

....

....

Motivation

Are you looking for a short-term or a long-term solution? As already mentioned, this book isn't for those looking to lose weight within a set period of time, it's for the realistic person who is fed up of living a life restricted by the way they look and feelings of unhappiness.

Your motivation for losing weight is key to your success, so let's revisit the above questions and look again at answering them with complete honesty.

Why should you make the changes within your life?

....

....

What happens if you fail to change your eating habits?

....

....

How will your life improve by eating nutritionally rich foods?

....

....

What will you do with your improved and increased energy?

....

....

What positive aspects of this change will be reflected in your loved ones?

....

....

Why is now the right time to make these massive changes?

....

....

Do you deserve to be fit, healthy and happy?

....

....

Why will you never go back to being the way you were?

....

....

"Life is 10% what happens to me and 90% how I react to it." -
Charles Swindoll

Skinny-Fat And Fat-Fat, DON'T Be Fooled

Okay, fat reality check time. We now know what fat is on a
nutritional level but it's time to consider what it is in relation to the
size of a person. There are many factors to be considered here. For
example, someone who is six feet tall and weighs 13 stone is going
to look very different to someone who weighs the same but is only
five feet tall. Weight and fat are two completely different aspects of
size yet weight seems to be considered the overall deciding factor by
most when it comes to health.

The common assumption is that a heavy person must be a fat
person but there's more to fat than just weight.

Skinny-fat – this describes the person who rarely eats, fails to
exercise, and generally speaking will be a smoker in a stressful job
(often in sales or accounting) with a dependant family at home.
They are skinny but they hold more body fat than muscle, and
the lack of quality nutrition actually causes a lack of growth and
therefore skinniness. They are effectively functioning on the
minimum levels of nutritional value, generally sourced through a
diet of foods low in protein and carbohydrate, and high in saturated

fats.

Fat-fat – this describes the person who consumes too much and does too little in terms of physical exercise. Generally speaking, they adopt a lazy attitude to most things in life, other than things of immediate interest, and this leads to a failure to recognise the importance of nutrition and its effect on their overall health and wellbeing. In most cases, a fat-fat person will stick to the minimum nutritional guidelines set out by the government and they will often use 'genetics' as a reason for being the way they are.

I feel it's important to mention this now because people often arrive at my seminars with preconceived ideas concerning size. The ultimate aim is to shift your focus away from skinny versus fat to see a fat-neutral state as the way forward in terms of health as well as self-perception. We need fat to live and we also need muscle so aiming to sit nicely between skinny and fat is the way to begin enjoying being in your body.

How much fat would I be happy with on my body?

....

....

How much fat is too much?

....

....

How can I achieve a fat-neutral self-perception?

....

....

Why Do You Want To Lose Weight – Please Be Honest!

Vanity – if you are looking to lose weight simply for vanity reasons, then here is the shocker: over 90% of my clients who lie when they answer the question of *why* end up back where they started. They have a goal, they lose weight – they then flip back to old habits and put the weight back on. Losing weight to change the way you look is a big motivator but it's important not to let it be the main reason. It's a big temptation, but by focusing on the way you look you run the risk of achieving your ideal look, being happy with it, and then forgetting everything you learned on your journey to get there.

Trying to fit in – another temptation to avoid is making changes to your diet simply to fit in with the current trend. This is increasingly popular in modern culture as social media helps to spread the word on the latest celebrity endorsed new (which really just means re-branded) diet. The moment an airbrushed celebrity shares "the secret" of their instant and fabulous new look, people are very quick to jump on the bandwagon – believing the same instant results will be theirs.

Trending diets have been around for the last 80 years and the number of 'new' diets appears to be increasing daily. Of course, we can't deny the evolution of medicine and science and the fact that we're still learning new concepts, but let's just think about the last 20 years or so and make some clear observations:

Obesity rates are climbing daily

It is reported that obesity and related illnesses will bankrupt the NHS by 2022

Fast food is becoming a staple in the majority of daily diets

Jobs involving physical labour are decreasing as the use of technology is increasing

The population is increasing and living space is decreasing

Home economics is no longer taught in most schools

Children are no longer participating in daily sports or outdoor activities.

Expectations to perform at higher levels for extended times.

These are just a few observations but when looked at collectively, the reason why we have these issues stands out. Avoid the temptation to follow a trend; the information contained within this book is a cut back and functional solution to get your diet back on track and achieve the results you want – no frills, just simple and honest advice.

To please another – this is a tricky subject that comes up frequently during my female one-to-one sessions. Changing the way you look to please another isn't going to deliver the results you think it will. The change has to come from within you and for your own reasons, not the reasons of another.

"Your time is limited; so don't waste it living someone else's life."
– Steve Jobs

If you're having relationship issues because of a partner's behaviour and attitude to your weight, then avoid the belief that losing weight will change those behaviours. Losing weight *will* change your behaviour as you gain greater self-confidence but you must also address the reaction from your partner – has anything really changed? This is a subject that could fill a book of its own so, for now, take my advice and change because *you* want to, not because someone else tells you to.

TASK

Grab a pen and write down five top reasons why you should lose weight. Mix up the answers with both long and short-term objectives. Keep the language used positive and avoid the temptation to over exaggerate.

....

....

....

....

....

....

Exercise

As already mentioned, and in simplistic terms, energy that isn't used will be stored as fat. The human body is designed to move but with modern living no longer requiring the same degree of physical effort and daily tasks no longer as labour intensive as they once were, we need to make a conscious effort to introduce movement into our lives.

For those who don't currently partake in it, exercise is generally thought of as something that induces aches and pains and requires hours of sweating over something each week. Exercise is seen as a chore but in truth it can be so much more. The act of movement can be anything from a daily walk to work, to circuits/classes, to dancing or tennis, or any other activity at all that gets you moving.

A lack of exercise causes endless issues on both a physical and mental level. Movement aids digestion and helps to cleanse the body as well as generating the release of essential mood enhancing chemicals that simulate positive thinking and performance.

What can you implement right now that will increase the movement within your life?

....

....

How much time can you commit every day to additional movement?

....

....

What You Should Be Doing

There are many different types of exercise programmes on the market, all with unique benefits and designed to suit a variety of fitness levels. Having worked with many hundreds of people, I have altered and adapted my programmes to engage each aspect of the body while increasing the cardiovascular capacity.

I've included two of the most popular programmes below and you can use them as often as you wish. However, the people who report the best results tend to take part in some form of activity at least three times a week, gradually increasing to five. At the back of the book I've included an explanation of each of the exercises, but they can also be found online.

Added note: there is no substitute to training as part of a group. Being in the company of others very often boosts motivation, increasing the ability of all concerned, and it provides accountability. However, I do appreciate that not everyone has the opportunity or the resources to attend a club or gym.

When completing the exercises below, the aim is to raise your breathing rate to the point that you can just about hold a conversation, but your sentences are becoming shorter! Make sure you have enough room around you and only start when it's safe to do so.

BOOTCAMP WORKOUT # 1

Warm Up – 1 Minute of Running on the Spot

1.	Lunges Alternate	24 Reps
2.	Squats	24 Reps
3.	Lunge to Rotation	24 Reps
4.	Squat Jumps	12 Reps
5.	Hold the Plank	30 seconds

30 Second Rest

6.	Press Ups Narrow Seconds Rest	50 Seconds Exercise, 10
7.	Press Ups Normal Seconds Rest	50 Seconds Exercise, 10
8.	Press Ups Staggered Seconds Rest	50 Seconds Exercise, 10
9.	Press Ups Hands Out Seconds Rest	50 Seconds Exercise, 10
10.	Bent Over Rows Seconds Rest	50 Seconds Exercise, 10
11.	Shoulder press Seconds Rest	50 Seconds Exercise, 10
12.	Upright Row/ Lateral Raise	50 Seconds Exercise, 10

Seconds Rest

13. Bicep Curls   50 Seconds Exercise, 10
    Seconds Rest
14. Triceps Extensions   50 Seconds Exercise, 10
    Seconds Rest

Sprint on the Spot – 20 seconds on 20 seconds off 20 seconds on. Rest 20 seconds then repeat twice.

15. Crawl Outs   30 Seconds Exercise, 15
    Seconds Rest
16. Burpees   30 Seconds Exercise, 30
    Seconds Rest

High Knees – 20 seconds on 20 seconds off 20 seconds on. Rest 20 seconds then repeat twice.

17. Crunches   50 Seconds Exercise, 10
    Seconds Rest
18. Obliques   50 Seconds Exercise, 10
    Seconds Rest
19. Reverse Curls   50 Seconds Exercise, 10
    Seconds Rest
20. Cross Overs   50 Seconds Exercise, 10
    Seconds Rest
21. Bicycle   50 Seconds Exercise, 10
    Seconds Rest
22. Kick Outs   16, 12, 8, 4, 2 slow, 1 hold
    for 10 seconds, 10 fast (each side)
23. Plank to Press Up   50 Seconds Exercise, 10
    Seconds Rest
24. Side Plank   50 Seconds Exercise, 10
    Seconds Rest
25. Squat Thrusts   50 Seconds Exercise, 10
    Seconds Rest

BOOTCAMP WORKOUT # 2

Warm Up – 1 Minute of Running on the Spot

30 Second Rest

1. Lunges Alternate   24 Reps
2. Squats   24 Reps
3. Lunge to Rotation   24 Reps
4. Squat Jumps   12 Reps
5. Hold the Plank   30 Seconds

30 Second Rest

Ladders – 3 Exercises in Each Ladder Drill 1-10 Reps of Each Then Back Down From 10-1

6. Bent Over Rows
7. Shoulder Press
8. Bicep Curls

1-10 Reps of Each Then Back Down From 10-1

9. Press Ups
10. Squats – holding weight between legs
11. Triceps Extensions

1-10 Reps of Each Then Back Down From 10-1

12. Squats
13. Burpees
14. Crunches

1-10 Reps of Each Then Back Down From 10-1

15. Obliques (each side)
16. Reverse Curls
17. Hip Raises

Cardio Circuit

18. Sprint on the Spot   50 Seconds Exercise, 10
Seconds Rest

19. High Knees   50 Seconds Exercise, 10
Seconds Rest

20. Heel Flicks   50 Seconds Exercise, 10
Seconds Rest

21. Crawl Outs   50 Seconds Exercise, 10
Seconds Rest

22. Side Jumps   50 Seconds Exercise, 10
Seconds Rest

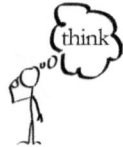

When can you commit to one of the above?

Day............................Time........................

Why is now the right time to set this?

....

....

How are you going to ensure that nothing interrupts this time?

....

....

CHAPTER FOUR

Nutrition – You Are What You Eat

It's time you started thinking for yourself and stopped accepting the past as guidance for the future.

Mass society teaches/educates us that everything must go through a process before it can be consumed hence the reason why more space is allocated to packaged items than fresh produce in our supermarkets. This accepted view needs to be changed and a more positive 'shopping focus' put in place. Another positive shift in thinking is to let go of the belief that a 'real' meal has to be served hot.

Do You Need Organic/Raw?

My own diet is varied and where possible I attempt to consume at least 90% organic foods. The organic food diet was alien to me at first, as with many people, and psychologically it offered many challenges. But, the more I began to understand the dynamics and science of how food is digested, the more I accepted that this was a solution offering everything my previous diet had been lacking.

There are many good reasons to eat organic foods and there are also good reasons to reduce the amount of food you cook. I'm not saying you should eat everything raw but the nutritional benefits it brings include aiding weight loss and the repairing of your body.

Eating quality food is great, but preparing it to get the maximum nutritional return is what really counts.

The organic raw food principle in a nutshell

(pun intended!): in the majority of cases, cooking a food decreases its nutritional value. As an example, vitamin C is destroyed by heat and the cancer-fighting properties of green vegetables such as broccoli are greatly diminished through cooking. It's for this reason that the bulk of a raw food diet is consumed in its raw state, and where cooking is required, temperatures remain below 48 degrees Celsius (118 degrees Fahrenheit) and ideally below 40 degrees Celsius (104 degrees Fahrenheit) to prevent heat damage and therefore preserve as much of the nutrient value as possible.

Think About This For A Moment ...

Visualise the journey a baked potato makes from field to fork. It begins in the ground, covered in earth and packed full of energy. It's uprooted and it begins its journey to the consumer. I'm unsure of the exact number of days it may be in transit or storage before making it to a shop shelf, and then the number of days it takes to journey from the shop shelf into a kitchen cupboard or fridge needs to be considered, let alone the time it may languish there before being used. The cooking process usually involves being baked in an oven at temperatures far greater than 40 degrees C to ensure the skin becomes dry and crispy before then smothering it in saturated fats to add moisture before consumption. Your body attempts to break down and extract any remaining nutrients but ultimately struggles due to the negative 'value' overload.

I know this is a slightly dramatic and overly simplified account of a baked potato's journey but the point I want to demonstrate is that sourcing any produce in its rawest of forms (dirt and all) and using it as quickly as possible in the rawest consumable way possible ensures the quality of the produce is transferred and fully utilised. Sure, a baked potato isn't a baked potato unless it goes through the baking process, however, this diet is not about eliminating essentially nutrient-dense foods from your diet, it's about understanding how altering the way you source and prepare food ultimately holds the key to getting the most nutritional value from the foods you eat.

I can guarantee that there is nothing more enjoyable than sitting down and eating something you have constructed and produced from scratch.

Food through new eyes — not something needed just to survive but something that creates a life worth living.

What changes can you make to your shopping habits?

....

....

Where can you source quality raw food?

....

....

Frozen Vs Fresh

Let The Debate Commence ...

There is no question that if you are able to source fresh produce then there really is no better option, however the fact remains that some ingredients are simply not geographically or physically possible to obtain fresh from source so rather than removing them completely from your diet, settling for frozen is the next best option.

In situations where you are unable to go directly to source, or foods are so far removed from being fresh after travelling thousands of miles over several days or perhaps weeks, then I would prefer to opt for the frozen version, especially if frozen at source. Why? As a general rule of thumb, fruits picked for freezing are usually processed prior to ripening, and, as this is when they usually display the peak level of nutritional value, the frozen version therefore represents a better choice than the 'fresh' version languishing on a supermarket shelf.

Of course, there are mixed opinions on this subject and the debate will no doubt rumble on and continue to waste more energy than needed, but let's just use the potato example once more. I am fortunate to have a farm shop less than a few miles from my home and I know that the potatoes sold there are certainly sourced from within a reasonable distance of the shop and 100% from within the UK. However, a quick look at the prepackaged options available in most of the larger grocery stores nationwide will reveal that many varieties are imported.

It makes perfect sense to buy as fresh as possible. When foods are exposed to excessive heat and light after being uprooted from their natural state, the nutrients begin to degrade significantly, especially vitamin C and thiamin (vitamin B) which are particularly delicate. The balance therefore becomes a matter of limiting the number of degenerative processes in order to maintain the highest possible nutrient value.

If you have decided that it's not going to be possible to source certain products from fresh then keep in mind that a frozen product should remain frozen until it's ready to be used. Thawing and re-freezing has a detrimental (sometimes potentially dangerous) effect on foods so items should only be thawed ready for immediate use. If you've ever re-frozen chocolate, you'll have noticed the whitening effect this has on its appearance, giving you an insight into the detrimental effect this could have on other produce.

Preparing The Feast – Eye Candy?

Sometimes more can be said for the way something looks than the way it tastes. If it looks good then the likelihood is it will taste good, or at least that's what the mind is attempting to process (via its senses), and this is exactly the tactic employed by marketing companies on food packaging. Ask yourself this: when was the last time a packaged meal actually turned out looking like it did on the packet? I'm pretty sure the answer is NEVER, and the reason for this is simple – it can't.

The first time I went into a wholefood store, the vibrant colours that glared back at me blinded me. This is a statement that can only be made subject to your past learnings. Let me explain: the mind, seeing something bright in colour, will associate what it sees with certain beliefs usually installed back in childhood. This can then go two ways, depending entirely on your childhood experiences of brightly coloured foods. If bright equated to good in your childhood, your mind will see vibrant foods as good foods, but if bright equated to bad in your childhood, your mind will see vibrant foods as bad foods.

For many years, food for me was something I needed to survive, not something I felt particularly inspired to spend any time on. I was fortunate with the foods I was given in my childhood, but eating food was still only considered to be a necessity and not an enjoyable part of life. Having fun with the colours you have available is essential, not only in your own food preparation but also in terms of showing others, the younger generations included, that **food = fun**.

The more we educate ourselves and others on food production and evolution, the more able we are to use food to our advantage and to create a strong respectful connection to the benefits.

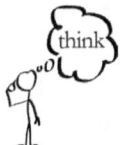

How can you improve the quality of the preparation?

....

....

What value do you attach to food?

....

....

In what ways have your food choices changed since starting the book?

....

....

Is Fresh The Solution?

The more appetising a food looks the more likely you are to eat it. Just think for a moment about the vast number of fast food outlets and the pictures they display of the 'meal deals' they have on offer – how often does the actual product look anything like the picture? Rarely: and if it did, I'd question the level of synthetic content required to create such an appearance.

The truth is that we primarily gauge our food choices on the visual representation along with the smell. It's only once we have satisfied these criteria that we consider the taste and texture. By using a hidden creative ability that we all have, we can think about preparing food as if preparing the paint to create a masterpiece.

So, let's quickly summarise the nutritionally rich foods you *can* eat at this point before you slip into focusing on what you *can't* eat. Nutritionally rich foods generally fall into the following factors.

Foods that represent their original state – be aware of products that have been refined to improve their appearance.

Foods that do not have any additional artificial flavours or colourings – this is because naturally nutritious foods don't need to have anything added to them.

Foods that are not packaged in a way to stop them from breaking down or following their own natural cycle - if it's rotten then it's rotten, simple.

Foods that have only one ingredient – a carrot is a carrot, no other ingredients should be listed.

Foods that don't have any sugars or refined white/bleached chemicals added – this is because they are good enough on their own.

The following foods are now staples in my own diet:

Salad vegetables, such as cucumbers and red onion
Salad toppings, such as olives
Garlic
Avocados
LOTS of cannellini beans
LOTS of rolled oats
LOTS of lentils
Other varieties of beans – black beans, pinto beans, garbanzo beans, etc.
Brown rice
Quinoa
Raisins
Soy and almond milk
Tofu
Canned tomatoes, crushed or diced
Salsa
Frozen fruit
Frozen vegetables
Balsamic vinegar
Nutritional yeast

Spices – curry powder, seasoning, chili powder, etc.
Maple syrup
Vegan vegetable bouillon

This basic diet consists of nuts, seeds, fruit (both fresh and dried), natural sweeteners, oils, vegetables, spices and herbs, salts and natural flavourings, and as the sample recipes on the following pages demonstrate, the seemingly limited food choices in no way limit the potential to create delicious and nutritious meals.

Getting Back To The Basics Of Living ...

If You Can't Pronounce It You Shouldn't Be Eating It

I think that by stripping back the ingredients to the rawest possible form, you not only simplify the overall process, you also make it much simpler to tailor your consumption needs to the type of lifestyle you live.

The basic concept with all nutrition is that you are simply a by-product of what you eat. The more time you spend re-educating yourself in terms of looking into which foods will support you in the best way possible, the more you make it possible to become a better version of yourself – the best version it's possible to be.

Why wouldn't you be the best you can be?

....

....

Why would you settle for anything less than great in life?

....

With nutrition, you have to ask yourself what is truly important: are you likely to love a better, healthier life consuming good, nutritionally rich foods, or a life plagued with illness and poison? This may seem like an overly stark comparison but the reality is that the more basic you become with your diet the better and healthier it's likely to be.

To really get back to basics, it's a good idea to adopt a 'baby mind'. When we are young, our vocabulary is limited and as we grow it expands and grows accordingly. In terms of diet, the more we grow the more experiences we gain of colours, tastes and textures so our food vocabulary also becomes more varied and colourful. When you use your baby mind, you go back to thinking about the words a baby might use to describe the food they want. In most cases, the foods a baby is aware of are healthy choices, and although limited, they represent foods that promote healthy living. It's only when we become adults that our mind takes on a belief structure of trusting others to provide truthful facts about the contents of food products and we trust that foods will not be labelled in such a way that any negative aspects are deliberately hidden from us as the consumer.

> 'Baby mind' foods might include: apple, peach, carrot, juice etc. After all, it's very unlikely that a baby would request a microwave meal topped with extra cheese and a side order of fries, isn't it?

On the subject of children, I make a very conscious effort as a parent and uncle to impartially educate children on the rights and wrongs of the world. One afternoon, while we were having a BBQ, a friend made a point of offering to take the children to a well-known fast food outlet for burgers, chips and a toy if they behaved. My son, Joseph (aged 9), confidently announced, "Shouldn't we be going somewhere that offers good food to reward us, not processed junk?"

Sure, it's fair to say that this way of thinking isn't the norm and, in fact, the majority of adults present laughed, but it's also fair to say that Joseph made a valid point. Within our culture we are taught that cake, chocolate and all things high in saturated fat are indeed a treat.

From this point forward change your thinking – think 'baby mind'.

Kitchen Basics

Okay, so what about the kitchen basics you'll need to make the most of your new and supportive diet! Remember, there's nothing complicated about the foods you'll be eating so there's no need for any complicated kitchen gadgetry.

There's every chance that everything you need is already in your kitchen. The basics are:

Knife – you'll need a sharp knife that can be used to chop everything from a pineapple to a bunch of fresh herbs. Make sure it can be cleaned and sharpened easily.

Chopping board – you'll need a quality board that will allow you to chop a wide variety of vegetables and fresh ingredients safely and easily. There are plenty of different styles and brands on the market so it comes down to personal choice. Fans of wooden boards believe wood has antibacterial properties and it won't dull your knife as quickly as plastic, but fans of plastic believe that being able to put your chopping board in the dishwasher makes it the most convenient option.

Measuring tools – you'll need a means of measuring out ingredients when following recipes. There are lots of simple and inexpensive options available in shops or you can just use utensils you already have in your kitchen. The key is to have designating measuring tools that will allow you to be consistent with your measurements.

Scrubbing brush – you'll need a brush that's robust enough to allow you to scrub soil etc. from fresh produce.

Blender, Juicer, Food processor, Dehydrator – Optional

The First Step

Like any new adventure, it can be both challenging and daunting when you begin looking for solutions, especially if you are the only one taking this path. Personally, I have found that you will meet two different types of people along the way: those who are interested and wish you luck, or those who will laugh in your face – literally. To overcome these minor confrontations, simply remember the deeper reason behind what you are planning to do and remind yourself of the long-term benefits of doing what you are doing.

Why are you improving your dietary habits?

....

....

Why is now the right time to change for the better?

....

....

What excuses have you made in the past?

....

....

Getting started at the store is going to be easier than you think. When I first started, I was keen to clear out the old and introduce the new, but the truth is that if you have been eating a relatively balanced diet then there is little that will go to waste. Sure, there are going to be lots of new and exciting additions but, overall, the changes are not as vast as one might assume.

On the topic of getting started, avoid making the assumption that it is going to be more expensive to eat raw foods or a diet consisting mainly of organic related produce. This is not actually true as eating more of the 'good stuff' is actually more cost effective in the majority of cases, even when organic produce is the primary choice. Sure, choosing organic varieties of everything may increase your costs depending on your location, but with a little research and perhaps organising a monthly rather than weekly shop, you can justify travelling slightly further afield to find better value in farm shops or farmers' markets. For example: I usually travel 10 miles to a rural farm shop to source all vegetables. These are bought in five and 10 kilo bags with a 10 kilo bag of carrots currently costing just under £3.00. Compare this to the £1.75 I'd need to pay for just one kilo in my local supermarket and that's a whooping saving of £14.50 in just one product.

Get Local

As previously mentioned, the closer you are to the source the finer the nutritional content, and as my own experiences show, costs can also be significantly reduced. Personally, I believe that buying locally is a winner all around, and better than so-called organics that are being imported from around the world. Investing in your local farmers allows them to invest in better farming methods and thus create a healthier product. I know that a visit to your local farmer may not be your solution but, where possible, always buy local.

Once you have sourced your 'natural consumables', it's time to look at the things that are simply unavailable locally. In the absence of a local health food store, the Internet offers a useful substitute, and once you have established a regular shopping list, costs can be lowered by buying in bulk. However, if you do have a natural/ health food store in your area that doesn't appear to stock the items you want, don't be afraid to ask because they may be willing to buy them in for you.

Stop Talking About It And Start Doing It

My pet hate, apart from someone failing to replace a toilet roll, is people failing to do what they start out to do. Personally, I think it shows the strength of a person (or lack of it), especially when they give up very shortly after starting. However, I am *not* saying that you should continue to run a marathon with an injury, but simply that when committing to change you have to follow it through.

How complicated is it to eat right?

....

....

The answer is that it's only as complicated as you choose to make it.

> *The biggest reason why people don't change their diet is that they have to take responsibility for their actions – and this is something that scares them.*

There are endless 'reasons' why we give up in certain situations …

Self-reflection has obviously played an important part of your journey thus far, hence the reason why you are reading this right now. So, thinking that things are too hard or denying yourself the opportunity to succeed by thinking, "This will never work for me," is natural, but the thoughts in your head directly influence the actions you take and therefore the outcomes you experience in your reality. If you think it's too hard, it is; if you think it won't work for you, it won't. With this in mind, it's the steps you take to overcome this negative mindset that makes the difference between making changes for the better or staying where you are.

"Whatever the mind of man can conceive and believe, it can achieve." **– Napoleon Hill**

Think about it for a moment; when you're in the gym, have you ever noticed that some people get on the treadmill every day and continue to do the same thing day in and day out for no apparent gain? They keep going but very little change appears to be happening, so why is this? Well, the bottom line is that they're failing to take the steps needed to generate positive change. They run, and then they eat fat, so they then run again, and then they eat fat again … and so it goes on, but nothing actually changes. They're stuck in that vicious cycle and getting nowhere. Continuing to do the same things will continue to bring you the same results – are the things you're doing now bringing you the results you want?

Also, I know I've mentioned this previously but think about food packaging and labelling; anything that can be considered a remotely 'healthy' option will be proudly advertised on the packaging. But here's the thing – anything that's a truly healthy option won't come with a wrapper that tells you so. We all know that something that sounds too good to be true probably isn't true (e.g. this packet contains delicious sticky toffee pudding and only three calories) but yet we tend to believe what we're told when we read information on packaged foods produced by well-known and respected food manufacturers.

To break away from this pattern of believing what you read,

remember that food manufacturers are business people and they're in the business of making money just like any other business. A good business is one that sustains employment and has the ability to grow and increase profit margins – the food manufacturing business is no different. It's for this reason that the only way to be sure of what you're eating is to prepare your own foods from scratch, preferably from their raw state. The more processes a food product has been through, the less nutritional value it will contain – simple.

Let's face it; we can all come up with any number of reasons why we'll never achieve whatever it is we want, and we can spend days, hours and even years looking back at where things went wrong or where things all just seemed a little bit too hard, but, trust me, if you commit to changing your diet today, it's never too late to achieve the life you want. Choose to eat the foods that represent the colourful, vibrant life you want to live.

The colours of your food represent the type of life you will live – dark, dull, flat, and toxic, or bright, shapely, and packed full of energy.

Okay, we've established that you really are a by-product of the foods you eat so now it's time to focus on the amount of food you should be eating. Once again, this is really nothing more than common sense, but we know that common sense doesn't always prevail.

Remember, eating right is only as complicated as you choose to make it. Eating the right amount of food doesn't need to be complicated – if it looks a lot then it probably is, and that's it. If the food on your plate is piled high and/or spilling over the edges, then the likelihood is you're over consuming. If you can see empty space around the edge of your plate and your food is relatively flat, rather than piled high in the centre, then you can be fairly sure you're on the right track.

When it comes to making good food choices, I like to use the phrase, "If a rabbit can eat it then so can I" but another phrase I keep in the back of my mind is, "You never see a skinny rabbit." The relevance of this is that the amount of food you eat is just as important as the types of food you eat in terms of eating a healthy diet. Just because a food is fresh, vibrant and healthy does not mean that you can eat as much of it as you want, and it's a fact that you can still become obese on a vegan/vegetarian diet.

It must also be remembered that the same principle applies to drinks in your diet. Only water and natural juices should be consumed, and fizzy, chemical-rich pops should be avoided. Personally, my liquid consumption now consists only of homemade juices, my own brand of protein powder shakes, coffee, and unlimited amounts of water.

Fact: if you **EAT FAT** you **GET FAT**

Hard fact: those who consume a poor diet are more likely to suffer from long-term negative emotional conditions.

Start looking in the right place ... something that never ceases to amaze me is the way that many high street stores effectively hide genuinely healthy foods. Just the other day, I was looking for the vegan/vegetarian section in a popular store and I eventually found it in-between the pharmacy and the pre-cooked meat deli. Now, not only does this not make any sense, it confirms my belief that larger corporations don't actually want to promote genuinely healthy eating. You see, they don't want to promote natural super-foods when there's far more money to be made from promoting packaged (highly processed) foods that proudly proclaim they're the 'healthy option' on the label. This isn't a witch-hunt; you can make up your own mind when you next go out shopping. Just try looking for the genuinely healthy foods on the shelves and see how much longer it takes you.

> **Interesting note**: a 2013 British Nutritional Foundation study revealed that almost one third of primary school pupils in the UK think that cheese is made from plants, and one quarter think that fish

fingers come from chicken or pigs. The study also
revealed that nearly one in 10 secondary school pupils
think that tomatoes grow underground, and that
there's confusion over the source of many diet staples
such as pasta and bread with many younger pupils
stating they believed them to be made from meat.

Re-education, re-education, re-education … commit to
exploring and accepting anything that will make you a better
person. It doesn't have to be 'trendy' and it doesn't have to be right
for the guy next door, it only has to be right for you. Any change
you make that brings even just one tiny positive aspect with it is a
change that's worth it.

CHAPTER FIVE

Food – More Than Just Food

Just remember the old adage, *"You are what you eat,"* and you won't go far wrong.

Consuming quality food becomes even more essential, if not critically so, when you are ill or struggling with chronic feelings of being under the weather. Becoming better at something means taking steps to learn how to improve and therefore do better in that something, right? Learning how to feel better through learning how to eat better is no different. The better your understanding of food and its effects on your body – both emotionally and physically – the stronger a position you put yourself in to be able to take control and improve your mental and physical health.

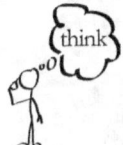

Think about this for a moment:

On a recent trip to a hospital, I was amazed by the types of foods being served in the canteens there, and not only that, but by the physical condition of those treating the ill. I estimate that an average of 80% of all the staff/medical professionals I witnessed were clinically obese... I consider someone to be obese if their knees rub together when they walk. Surely this doesn't make sense. We go to hospital to be treated because we are ill but while we're there we're fed rubbish – bland, colourless food – and we're treated by a number of professionals who apparently fail to take any notice of *their* industry recommendations.

Take a look at this NHS (National Health Service) report:

Being obese increases your risk of developing a number of serious and potentially life-threatening diseases, such as:

Type 2 diabetes
Heart disease
Some types of cancer, such as breast cancer and colon cancer
Stroke

In addition, obesity can damage your quality of life and can often trigger depression.

Source: http://www.nhs.uk

In my opinion, the above simply highlights the need for re-education in terms of the practical application of being able to eat, live and succeed, in the most vibrant and healthiest way possible.

Feed your life with HARD facts, not myths ... let's get real!

If you've reached this far in the book, the likelihood is that you have *really* identified that you need to change something... perhaps the pain has become unbearable, or perhaps you've simply identified that things can no longer continue as they are. Either way, movement is always good.

However, beware of self-affirmations during your dietary journey. Self-affirmations will either envelope you in a visualised reality or disassociate you from the truth. With food, it's usually the latter. When you disassociate yourself from the truth, you say things to yourself such as, "It doesn't matter," or, "Things will get better." You might also make strong, bold statements such as, "I will change in the New Year" or, "Just as soon as such and such has happened I'll change ..."

Of course, putting your head in the sand in such a way will almost always create a situation in which you inevitably become someone you could have avoided had you known the problems that would arise from these affirmations.

Ask yourself this: isn't it time you started living the life you always wanted?

Use affirmations, but ensure that they linguistically benefit you. The affirmations you use should move eating away from something that's a chore to something that's exciting. You control your life; it knows no boundaries other than those you give it. Allow it to run away with you and that's what will happen, but grasp it hard, control it and allow it to become something special… and it will.

What affirmation would inspire you to keep moving forward?

....

....

What additional education do you require in order to feel fully confident with your new journey?

....

....

Set yourself new goals based around what you have learnt thus far. Create a picture of a connection between food and a life boosting transformation beyond your wildest dreams, and avoid looking at food as something, which has brought about negative emotions in the past.

The Foods You Eat Vs. The Lifestyle You Live

Many times I talk with people who have been on any number of courses and training programmes or attended countless lectures and I'll always ask them to tell me in what way they've applied what they've learnt to their own lives. In over 70% of cases, they never have. They've gone on all of those courses yet they've failed to take action on anything they've learned. **Knowing** stuff is not enough, it's only by **applying** what you know that you can make change happen. Apply everything you have learnt so far and I can GUARANTEE that you will notice complete change in all aspects of your life.

"The world needs dreamers and the world needs doers. But above all, the world needs dreamers who do" – **Sarah Ban Breathnach**

> Only follow those who are practising what they preach. Something I have noticed A LOT within the FF industry (food and fitness industry) is that there are a great many people who tell but they don't apply: they talk the talk but they don't walk the walk. Only seek advice from those who have taken action to achieve what you want to achieve and therefore look like they actually believe in what they say.

It's my experience that a great many fitness instructors and dieticians don't look like they're taking their own advice. For this reason, whenever I'm looking for a mentor in some new adventure, I always look for a person who not only looks like they are doing as they say but also doing what they passionately believe in. I believe in my fitness programme and I'm constantly working towards improving it by making small adjustments along the way. Sometimes I learn through experience that there's a better way and I adjust my programme accordingly, and other times I learn that something is no longer effective and therefore I discard it. Either way, I'm constantly learning and I take what I learn forwards with me to ensure I continue to achieve the best results possible.

Stagnant programmes or thinking patterns will not evolve, and there are plenty of people out there selling products or programmes that are years out of date. Someone who truly believes in their message or product will be constantly moving and looking for ways to make improvements because they are 100% committed to delivering something of value – something that is constantly evolving. What I'm saying is that no matter what you're being told, make sure you're being told by someone who lives and breathes what he or she says and is highly committed to making themselves a better and stronger person. When you know that someone else has done it, you gain the motivation and confidence to do it for yourself, hence the reason why I would always where possible join a group or bootcamp to gain additional motivation, accountability and someone with the knowledge to guide you.

Where can you go that will support and help you where needed?

....

....

Who would you consider to be a suitable role model?

....

....

Reality Check

Okay, now is as good a time as any to pause, take a breath, and take a reality check. Throughout our lives, most of us accept that what is seen on the outside is predetermined by what is on the inside; we accept that who we are on the inside is reflected in the way we appear on the outside. So, how about flipping it? When working with clients in my practice, I ask them to consider and describe what the person on the inside is saying to person on the outside … and vice-versa.

In the majority of cases, the person on the inside will blame a number of emotions and past beliefs or experiences for the way they feel and the way they have acted as a result, meaning the way they have allowed themselves to form an unhealthy relationship with food. When we flip it and ask the person on the outside to describe the person on the inside, the focus more often than not switches away from the emotions and is placed on the physical and very *real* aspects of their life.

What we then have is two conflicting accounts of the 'truth'. A reality check is therefore essential and we have to break it down to discover the REAL TRUTH.

This process isn't solely focused on an individual's weight, but on their appearance, logic and overall health. The reality check helps to uncover the language each individual is using to describe themselves and the identity this gives them based on their overall appearance.

In other words, if you have become an unhealthy slob who consumes ready meals and gallons of fizzy pop then that's the appearance you will put out to the rest of the world – both the outer you and the inner you will reflect this identity. You can't lie about obesity or poor skin/health and the inner emotions you are experiencing will reveal the same truth.

How has the outside world seen you in the past?

....

....

What changes have you made so they don't see you like this in the future?

....

....

Why are you motivated to make these changes in your life right now?

....

....

So how will these changes appear when you improve your diet? The first change will be an internal change. It's likely that you'll go through a period of unrest initially until the clock is reset, but you'll then begin to feel the benefits of extended energy. You'll start to sleep better and as a result your complexion will change, and this leads into starting to feel more confident about your appearance. As this change happens, the language you use to describe yourself will also change and this is where the biggest impact occurs. By simply changing your diet, you change outwardly *and* inwardly and these changes provide the motivation to make larger lifestyle changes happens.

Now, there is a slight caveat: some people have reached a point of giving up internally and when this is the case they no longer care about their external appearance. They adopt an attitude of, "That's just the way I am," but this is tragic in my view. It is one thing to be accepting of your fate but it's quite another to limit your potential in life by resisting change and stubbornly refusing to adapt to doing things differently.

"I attribute my success to this: I never gave or took any excuse." –
Florence Nightingale

What can I do to ensure that I will not give up?

....

....

Moving forward, the life you live is only as good as you make it, right? Well, yes and no. It's certainly true that if you want to change your lot in life then you're going to have to take action to make those changes happen. But, as you become open to making changes, you will find there are plenty of people out there who are willing to offer their advice on just what changes you should make and many of your nearest and dearest will suddenly become diet and nutrition experts, all too willing to add their opinion to the mix. Change for the sake of change is not necessarily a good thing. Following the advice of 'experts' who clearly don't follow their own advice is unlikely to bring you the changes you want. You'll hear all sorts of things, and that's fine, but you need to know the exact direction you want to go in and the purpose of *your* adventure. When you're clear about the changes *you* want to see happen in your life, you're then in a position to discard any comments that are not relevant to you and the changes you want to achieve. Trust me, as soon as other people notice the positive changes in your complexion and they see that you're full of energy, they'll be asking *you* for your secrets and expert advice.

Tomorrow Is A Better Day ...

You are bound to experience a mass number of obstacles when changing anything. For me, the main obstacle was having lived a certain way for nearly 30 years and therefore having well-established habitual eating patterns. However, with each day of your new eating pattern, you begin to establish new habits and your old habits are soon left behind. I have met and worked with many people who have made this transition into healthy eating and as a result have transformed the way they act and live into a lifestyle that would previously only have been associated with someone many years their junior.

Nutrition, if you haven't guessed it already, is more than just the produce you put into your mouth, it's a whole new you; it's a whole new way of living and it's something you can use to better your life and extend your life. With this in mind, isn't it time you took back control of your life?

If you discovered you had cancer or diabetes and that your life was limited unless you made some changes right now this very moment, how long would you have to think about it before you committed to making those changes?

For most people, a switch to nutritionally good food can change their life around completely. As humans, we are fortunate to have the option of choice; the choice to do something or not, and in my world, that choice is just as important as the outcome. Out of all of the people I've worked with and helped to change all three pillars – lifestyle, nutrition and fitness – not one has ever asked me to help them change back to the person they were before. Why? Because we have choice, it's just that we tend to take our health for granted until it is too late.

Why wait for the change to happen? You have the ability to live a life as good as the healthiest person you know or as bad as the unhealthiest person you know, the deciding factor is nothing more than your choice. Only you can decide what you consume: factors such as money and geographic location can influence choices but they are rarely a valid reason for continuing to make poor choices.

"It is not necessary to change. Survival is not mandatory" – **W. Edwards Deming**

What Do You Value?

When asked to consider your response to being told you were suffering a terminal illness, it's my hope that this triggered some deeper realisations in terms of the actual value you place on your own life.

Through food, I have changed my value on life. Seeing through my own eyes how food and nutrition affects thinking as well as the physical body has been enough to ensure that I never, EVER, go back to the way I was. My value is knowing that I can always be better; that just because something didn't work in the past does not mean that it won't in the future, and that through consuming the right things I allow my body to work in the best possible form, thereby protecting me, supporting me, and allowing me to live the life I deserve.

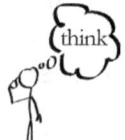

Why do you want your body to work in the best way possible?

....

....

What are you looking forward to doing with your new body?

....

....

Perhaps you're wondering how I can be so certain that I will never go back. Well, I'm certain because I've been around people grasping onto life; people who failed to take the action needed until it was too late; people who chose to abuse their bodies for years, and people who were consciously aware of doing wrong but only took heed of the damage being done once it had become too late. There are millions of people around the world suffering because of obesity and other dietary related illnesses and one thing is guaranteed; each one of them would turn back the clock and make a change if it meant they were able to spend just a few more days with loved ones, or perhaps be at a special event they will now miss.

The only time something becomes too late is when you fail to take the action when it comes into your mind for the first time. I call these the 'late lates' – a string of 'too lates' that then turn into later. Be aware of falling into this mindset. Putting things off for another time can be a slippery slope, especially if changing your diet is something you've thought about before but failed to take action on.

"Life is what happens to you while you're busy making other plans." – **John Lennon**

Remember, it doesn't matter what your motivations or reasons are, the most important thing is that you are doing it because you are fully aware of the health benefits associated with being healthy and the massive improvements it will bring to your lifestyle.

It's never too late… simple!

Remember the Art of Replacement

Have you ever been in a situation where you have given something up and all you can do is think about it? No matter what you do to distract yourself, the one thing you can't have is the one thing you want, right?

Smokers and dieters are among those who are most likely to experience this. Cigarettes and food are the only things they can think about as soon as they try to give them up. The reason for this is the relationship and close connection they have with these items. The things that attracted them into the relationship in the first place become the things they focus on when they can no longer have them, and the things they find themselves 'craving' and wanting back.

To rid yourself of these cravings and feelings of want you need to understand the art of replacement. Simply taking something away isn't going to work as this leaves a hole that needs to be filled – hence the craving. Replace the something that is taken away with something else fills the hole and curbs the craving, but the replacement must of course be a genuinely healthy option. Getting into the habit of doing without can be tough and it's for this reason that the art of replacement is likely to be much more effective in the long term as a new and positive habit is formed.

Have you ever tried to take an ice cream away from a baby, or a bone from a dog?

The subconscious mind is very clever at identifying things that are missing; the conscious skill is the art of replacing it until the new replacement is viewed as the better alternative.

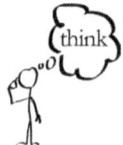

What challenges in the past can be replaced with something more positive in the future?

....

....

Isn't It Time You Started Listening to Your Body?

There are many reasons why you may already have started to change the way you eat and just as many for wanting to be able to change if you haven't started already. Each reason is unique to you and each is a valued reason I am sure, but one thing many of us within western culture have forgotten to do is to listen to our body.

We should all learn how to listen to our bodies and we should all then take the time to actually do it. Your body is really good at describing exactly what it needs. For example, think about the way you feel when you're thirsty ... your body lets you know it needs hydration. What about when you're hungry? Once again, your body lets you know it needs fuel; but what about when you're full? This question is not quite so straightforward to answer. The majority of us know when we're full so our bodies *do* let us know, the problem is that the majority of us fail to listen ... we continue to eat even though our bodies have signalled that we're full. We overeat because we choose to over-rule the signals that we're full in favour of continuing to gorge on the foods we mistakenly believe are making us feel good.

The human body has evolved to survive but, unfortunately, many of the people I meet are barely doing that. Through a general lack of understanding about nutrition, the diet many people 'survive' on today no longer fits into our evolutionary needs and the end result is obesity and the associated poor health issues. As a species we've become lazy, not only in our tendency to avoid exercise but also in our attitude to eating and our food choices.

"Life isn't about getting and having, it's about giving and being."
– Kevin Kruse

Important recap: you have absolute control over your journey in life. If you want to be sad, unhealthy and end up reducing your life by 10 or even more years then carry on. But, if you want to grasp life by the balls and make the most of every day, then you NEED to focus on re-educating yourself and gaining an understanding of nutrition and food. Change the focus away from what you can't have and what you can't do and place it on what you can have and what you can do. This change in thinking goes a long way towards improving the way in which you view food and this, in turn, gives you the ability to overcome any cravings you may have.

Negative people generally mix with negative people – it's called bonding through moaning – don't be one of them.

Top Tip: avoid where possible beating yourself up over eating a certain way in the past. You are now on the mend and taking steps to change your life for the better. Remember, it's not magic, it's just good eating. Commit to eating healthily at least 80% of the time and accept that the occasional chocolate bar (or similar) will not do *that* much harm.

You'll quickly notice that the more your body undergoes the transformation – releasing and letting go of those unwanted chemicals – you'll start to crave healthier, more beneficial ingredients in your daily diet. In fact, you'll very quickly notice that the majority of foods you once thought were packed full of flavour will become quite foul!

Get excited about the positive things this journey will bring as it's essential that you keep a positive mindset. The way you look at your nutrition and think about food has more of an effect than you may have realised. Positive thinking will now become more important than ever before and this includes loving your body from the outset. Starting to love and respect your body will in turn manifest into becoming a stronger person. Think about it this way; the more you love yourself, the more respect you will have for yourself, and the more you will consciously think about the foods you consume as a result.

You Only Live Twice

This title plays a significant role in my past and I'm certain it's one that many others can relate to. Within life, we can live one life with one diet and accept one path or we can grasp the opportunity to change it and live a second life. What we consume affects everything; how we act and feel changes the way we see the outside world. The changes in our diet can affect everything in our life – 55% of the way we communicate may be via physiology but 80% of how we perform is the result of what we consume.

The importance of diet cannot be stressed enough. If you fail to look after the factor that controls the majority of how you function, you will never reach your full potential. Accept that you have the opportunity to live twice – the old you and now the new you. Your second life is going to be the lifestyle you choose to maintain for the rest of your life, and choosing to make changes in the foods you consume now will allow you to finally be the person you have already dreamed of becoming.

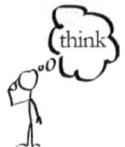

What is your life going to look like 10 years from now with your new changes?

....

....

What are you most excited about doing?

....

....

Time Vs. Benefits With Food Production

This is something I find highly frustrating, not solely because it's an excuse used by many people without thinking it through, but because it factually couldn't be any further than the truth. I can prepare a highly nutritional meal within half the amount of time it takes to microwave a meal and I can juice in half the time it takes to make a cup of coffee.

Time management may seem like a strange topic of discussion in relation to changing/ altering your diet, but if you are someone who is living a fast-pasted lifestyle then you're going to need some kind of routine and forward planning in place. The solution to any perceived time restraints is to prepare your meals the night before and use Tupperware. It couldn't be any easier. Nuts, seeds, beans, vegetables and even juices can all be prepared in advance and stored ready for the next day. Grabbing a pre-prepared pot is a lot faster than driving through your local fast food drive-thru or queuing at your local supermarket, in fact, when you think about it, there is nothing fast about fast-food. The only thing it's fast for is speeding up diet related illnesses.

I've mentioned a few times that improving your diet will lead to improvements in your energy levels. This is not a myth, or something made up by 'fitties' to annoy 'fatties', it's a fact. Think about the logic behind it; vegetables and all things natural absorb energy from the outside world and use it for growth. We can then utilise it and transfer it into our bodies through digestion.

Use linguistics to look at food differently – start using words such as dirty, poor, nasty or disgusting to repel any positive connections with processed products.

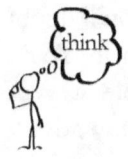

Why is dedicating the right amount of time to a diet key in your future?

....

....

How much time are you committing to improving the quality of your life?

....

....

Why is this important?

....

....

How and where can you overcome any obstacles?

....

....

Challenges – How Are You Going to Get Over Them?

As with any form of change, you will meet a whole host of different challenges along the way. You'll be subjected to criticism, you'll doubt yourself, and you'll even start to wonder if it's all worth it. You'll perhaps come up with a number of reasons why your old way of life was better, but I can promise you that if you follow my advice with 100% commitment and focus, you'll be able to make positive changes to your diet that last a lifetime. You won't want to go back to your old ways and who knows, you'll perhaps start to make changes in other areas of your life.

Habits take time to change, but avoid the temptation to slip into a false sense of security. Be honest from the very beginning and you'll see results appears a lot faster than you would if you were to stay within the security of the unhappiness that you're experiencing at the moment.

It's all about tomorrow – so many people I know want to know the shortcut to losing those additional pounds in body fat or how to get a six-pack within two weeks. The only shortcut to any of these things is to take action today so that tomorrow will be a lesser challenge. We would all love to be able to change our diet overnight and wake up looking like an Adonis in the morning but it's not going to happen. Committing to making changes in your diet will get you 80% of the way towards being your 'best you' but the other two factors of lifestyle and fitness must be addressed in order to get you all the way there.

Getting the Family on the Healthy Eating Team

You'd think it would be easy to get partners and spouses on board but it has been my experience that family members can be the biggest cynics of them all. This is especially true if they have seen you 'try' something new in past only to have given up when things weren't quite going the way you hoped. I have no shame in admitting that I have been that person.

What I am getting at is that no matter how highly motivated you may be, there's no guarantee that those around you will share your passion. However, if you are a parent, you can share your enthusiasm with your children and positively influence their food choices. If you are changing your diet for the better then by default you should be changing your children's diet for the better.

I love food and share my experiences where I can; food is my daily celebration and reward.

Each New Year, it makes me laugh to see overweight adults out buying up every new slimming product on the market yet continuing to buy the same old junk foods for their children. Does it make sense to improve your own diet but feed those you love the most the foods that led to you being unhappy and buying up slimming products in desperation? No!

My recommendation is to start gently with children by introducing them to the fun aspects of food. You'll get a much better buy-in if they are having fun experimenting with new foods rather than being told it's something they must do. Keep your whole family healthy by only buying nutritionally rich food and keeping your kitchen cupboards free of any nutritionally poor options. An easy motto to go by is – *If it's not in the house then I can't eat it.*

CHAPTER SIX

Recipes

Now that we've covered the thinking, values and purposes of food, you will hopefully have changed the way in which you view the basics of your dietary requirements. Over the next few pages I've included some recipes for really tasty and interesting dishes. There are plenty to give you variety but not so many that you become bewildered by choices. Each one is quick to prepare and nutritionally rich in protein, carbohydrates, fats and minerals. They are designed to kick-start a cleansing process, enabling you to start building a diet based on the food choices you are likely to consume in the future. Some of the ingredients may be new to you, perhaps even slightly alien, but all I ask is that you give them a try and then make adaptations to suit your palette.

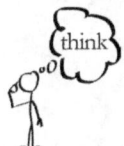

Think for a moment; how many different types of meals do you consume on a weekly basis?

....

....

How often do you change your breakfast?

....

....

What can you do to overcome any mindful objections when making these meals?

....

What is the reason behind changing your diet?

....

....

5 Healthy Breakfasts

Healthy Breakfast Number 1

Banana & Almond Butter Toast

Ingredients

    1 tablespoon almond butter
    1 slice rye bread, toasted
    1 banana, sliced

Directions:

1. Spread almond butter on toast.

2. Top with banana slices.

Healthy Breakfast Number 2

Honey Grapefruit with Banana

Ingredients

1 red grapefruit in sections (about 2 cups)
1 cup sliced banana (about 1)
1 tablespoon fresh chopped mint
1 tablespoon raw honey

Directions:

1. Combine grapefruit sections and remaining ingredients in a medium bowl. Toss gently to coat. Serve immediately, or cover and chill.

Healthy Breakfast Number 3

Spiced Green Tea Smoothie

Ingredients

3/4 cup strong green tea, chilled
1/8 teaspoon cayenne pepper
Juice of 1 lemon (2-3 tablespoons)
2 teaspoons agave nectar
1 small pear, skin on, cut into pieces
2 tablespoons fat-free plain yogurt
6-8 ice cubes

Directions:

1. Put all ingredients in blender. Blend until smooth. Drink cold.

Healthy Breakfast Number 4

Breakfast Barley with Banana & Sunflower Seeds

Ingredients

2/3 cup water

1/3 cup uncooked quick-cooking pearl barley

1 banana, sliced

1 tablespoon unsalted sunflower seeds

1 teaspoon honey

Directions:

1. Combine 2/3 cup water and barley in a saucepan, bring to boil and simmer.

2. Stir and let stand 2 minutes.

3. Top with banana slices, sunflower seeds, and honey.

Healthy Breakfast Number 5

Greek Yogurt Fruit Parfait

Ingredients

3/4 cup fat-free plain Greek yogurt

2 cups sliced mixed plums, peaches, and nectarines

3/4 cup puffed rice cereal (organic)

2 tablespoons walnuts and almonds, toasted and chopped

1 tablespoon ground flaxseed

1 tablespoon maple syrup, agave nectar, or honey

Directions:

1. In a tall 4-cup container or jar, layer half of the yogurt, fruit, cereal, nuts, flaxseed, and syrup. Repeat with the remaining half of ingredients, ending with syrup. (If you prefer a crunchy parfait, pack cereal separately to add right before eating.) Refrigerate up to 5 hours or overnight.

5 Healthy Lunches

Healthy Lunch Number 1

Broccoli Omelette with Toast

Ingredients

> Olive oil
> 1 cup chopped broccoli
> 2 large eggs, beaten
> 1/4 teaspoon dried dill
> 2 slices rye bread, toasted

Directions:

1. Heat a non-stick skillet over medium heat. Coat pan with olive oil. Add broccoli, and cook 3 minutes.

2. Combine egg and dill in a small bowl. Add egg mixture to pan. Cook 3 to 4 minutes; flip omelette and cook 2 minutes or until cooked through. Serve with toast.

Healthy Lunch Number 2

White Bean & Herb Hummus with Crudités

Ingredients

> 1/4 cup canned white beans, rinsed and drained
> 1 tablespoon chopped chives
> 1 tablespoon lemon juice
> 2 teaspoons olive oil
> Assorted raw vegetables, such as chopped broccoli florets, sliced green and red peppers, and baby carrots

Directions:

1. Combine beans, chives, lemon juice, and oil in a small bowl. Mash with a fork until smooth.

2. Serve with 1/2 cup raw vegetables, such as cucumbers, carrots, sugar snap peas, bell peppers, broccoli, and cherry tomatoes.

Healthy Lunch Number 3

Middle Eastern Rice Salad

Ingredients

2 tablespoons olive oil
1/2 sweet onion, thinly sliced (about 3/4 cup)
1 (16-ounce) can chickpeas, rinsed and drained
1/2 teaspoon ground cumin
1/4 teaspoon salt
Freshly ground black pepper
3 cups cooked brown rice
1/2 cup chopped pitted dates
1/4 cup chopped fresh mint
1/4 cup chopped fresh parsley

Directions:

1. Heat oil in a large non-stick skillet over medium-high heat. Add onion and cook, stirring often, about 5 minutes or until onion begins to brown. Remove from heat, and stir in chickpeas, cumin and salt. Season to taste with freshly ground black pepper.

2. Combine rice, onion-chickpea mixture, dates, mint, and parsley in a large bowl. Toss well until thoroughly combined. Serve warm or at room temperature.

Healthy Lunch Number 4

Energy-Revving Quinoa

Ingredients

    1 cup cooked quinoa
    1/3 cup canned low-sodium black beans, drained and rinsed
    1 small tomato, chopped
    1 scallion, sliced
    1 teaspoon olive oil
    1 teaspoon fresh lemon juice
    Pinch of salt
    Pinch of freshly ground black pepper

Directions:

    1. In a medium bowl, gently toss all ingredients to combine.

Healthy Lunch Number 5

Curried Egg Salad Sandwich

Ingredients

    2 hard-boiled eggs, chopped
    2 tablespoons plain Greek-style low-fat yogurt
    2 tablespoons chopped red bell pepper
    1/4 teaspoon curry powder
    1/8 teaspoon salt
    1/8 teaspoon pepper
    2 slices rye bread, toasted
    1/2 cup fresh spinach
    1 orange

Directions:

    1. Combine eggs, yogurt, bell pepper, curry powder, salt and
        pepper in a small bowl; stir well.

2. Place spinach on rye bread, top with egg salad, and serve the orange on the side.

10 Healthy Dinners

Healthy Dinner Number 1

Stir-Fry with Avocado Salad

Makes: 4 servings
Prep time: 10 minutes
Cook time: 10 minutes

Ingredients:

12 ounces beef tenderloin, cut into thin strips
1/4 cup freshly squeezed lime juice
1 tablespoon plus 1/2 teaspoon chilli powder
1 tablespoon olive oil
1 medium sweet onion, thinly sliced
1 red bell pepper, thinly sliced
1 poblano (mild chilli pepper), thinly sliced
1/2 teaspoon salt
1/2 teaspoon black pepper
1 can black beans, rinsed and drained
1 avocado, diced
1/4 cup coriander plus more for garnish, chopped

Directions:

1. In a bowl, combine beef, 2 tablespoons lime juice, and 1 tablespoon chilli powder; set aside.
2. Heat oil in a large skillet. Add onion, bell pepper, and poblano and sauté 5 minutes, stirring occasionally.
3. Add beef and marinade to vegetables and cook 3 to 4 minutes. Season with salt and black pepper.

4. In another bowl, combine beans, avocado, 1/4 cup coriander, and remaining lime juice and chilli powder.
5. Garnish beef and vegetables with remaining coriander. Serve with avocado salad and warmed tortillas if desired.

Healthy Dinner Number 2

Lemon-Thyme Chicken with Sautéed Vegetables

Makes: 4 servings
Prep time: 5 minutes
Cook time: 15 minutes

Ingredients:

4 tablespoons lemon juice
1 tablespoon chopped garlic, divided
1 tablespoon chopped fresh thyme, divided
Salt
Freshly ground black pepper
1 lb chicken breast fillets, lightly pounded
4 teaspoons olive oil
1 medium shallot, sliced
1 ½ cups frozen shelled edamame, thawed
1 ½ cups cherry tomatoes, halved
2 medium courgettes

Directions:

1. In a re-sealable plastic bag, combine 3 tablespoons lemon juice, 2 teaspoons garlic, and 2 teaspoons thyme; season to taste with salt and black pepper. Add chicken fillets, seal the bag, and gently turn to coat. Set aside.

2. Heat 2 teaspoons olive oil in a large skillet over medium-high heat. Add shallot, remaining garlic, edamame, and tomatoes; sauté 4 minutes.

3. Use a vegetable peeler to slice courgette into long ribbons. Add courgette and remaining lemon juice and thyme to vegetables in skillet; sauté 2 to 3 minutes. Transfer to a serving bowl, stir in feta, and season with salt and black pepper to taste.

4. Add remaining oil to skillet. Remove chicken from marinade and sauté 2 to 3 minutes a side or until cooked through. Serve with vegetables.

Healthy Dinner Number 3

Chilli Roasted Salmon

Makes: 4 servings
Prep time: 10 minutes
Cook time: 10 minutes

Ingredients

Olive Oil
4 tablespoons fresh lime juice
4 garlic cloves, smashed
2 teaspoons chilli powder
2 teaspoons ground cumin
3 teaspoons olive oil
4 5-ounce skinless salmon fillets
1 ½ cups frozen corn kernels (sweetcorn), thawed
1 red bell pepper, thinly sliced
1 poblano (mild chilli pepper), thinly sliced
1/2 small red onion, thinly sliced
Salt
Freshly ground black pepper
2 tablespoons chopped fresh coriander

Directions:

1. Preheat the oven to 220° C. Mist 2 large baking sheets with olive oil. In a small baking dish, mix together 2 tablespoons lime juice with garlic, chilli powder, cumin, and 1 teaspoon olive oil. Add salmon and turn to coat; let sit.

2. In a medium bowl, toss corn, bell pepper, poblano pepper, and onion with remaining 2 teaspoons olive oil. Transfer corn mixture to one of the baking sheets; spread into a single layer.

3. Remove salmon from marinade and arrange on second baking sheet. Drizzle corn mixture with remaining salmon marinade. Season salmon and corn with salt and black pepper to taste and roast 8 to 10 minutes, until fish is just cooked through and vegetables are tender.

4. Mix together coriander, and remaining lime juice. Season with salt to taste. Spoon corn onto plates and add salmon. Drizzle cream over fish.

Healthy Dinner Number 4

Mustard-Rubbed Pork Tenderloin with Brussels Sprout Ragout

Makes: 4 servings
Prep time: 5 minutes
Cook time: 20 minutes

Ingredients

> 10 ounces Brussels sprouts, quartered
> 3/4 teaspoon salt
> 3/4 teaspoon freshly ground black pepper
> 1 large pork tenderloin (about 1 ¼ lbs), butterflied
> 2 tablespoons Dijon mustard
> 2 tablespoons olive oil
> 1/4 cup white wine

1/4 cup chicken stock
1/2 cup diced pancetta or bacon
1 small yellow onion, thinly sliced
1/4 cup dried cherries
1 tablespoon chopped sage leaves

Directions:

1. In a medium pot fitted with a steamer, steam Brussels sprouts 8 minutes.

2. Sprinkle 1/2 teaspoon each salt and black pepper on pork and then spread with mustard. In a 12-inch skillet, warm 1 tablespoon olive oil over medium-high heat; add pork and cook 7 minutes. Turn and cook 6 minutes more; remove from pan and slice. Add wine and chicken stock to pan and stir, scraping up brown bits; set aside and keep warm.

3. Warm remaining olive oil in a small sauté pan over medium-high heat. Add pancetta or bacon and sauté until brown, stirring occasionally, about 3 minutes. Reduce heat to medium and add onion; cook until translucent, 5 minutes. Add cherries, sage, and Brussels sprouts; cook 3 minutes more. Season with remaining salt and black pepper.

4. On a platter, arrange pork and vegetables; drizzle with sauce. Serve.

Healthy Dinner Number 5

Chicken Soba Bowl

Makes: 4 servings
Prep time: 5 minutes
Cook time: 12 minutes

Ingredients

3 tablespoons orange juice
1 tablespoon lemon juice
1 tablespoon soy sauce
1 tablespoon sesame oil
1 pepper, seeded and minced
2 teaspoons minced lemongrass or lemon zest
1 teaspoon grated ginger
Salt
1 lb chicken fillets
6 ounces noodles
2 cups sliced fresh shiitake mushrooms, stems removed
4 baby bok choy (Chinese cabbage), quartered
3 cups broccoli florets
1/4 cup torn basil leaves (optional)

Directions:

1. In a large bowl, whisk together orange juice, lemon juice, soy sauce, sesame oil, pepper, lemongrass or lemon zest, and ginger.

2. Fill a large skillet 3/4 full with water, add a sprinkle of salt and bring to a simmer. Add chicken fillets and cook 5 to 7 minutes or until chicken is tender. Drain chicken and shred directly into bowl with dressing.

3. Bring a large pot of salted water to the boil. Add noodles and shiitakes; cook 3 minutes. Add bok choy and broccoli; cook 1 to 2 minutes or until noodles are al dente.

5. Drain noodles and vegetables and add to bowl with chicken and dressing. Toss gently to combine. Garnish with basil if desired.

Healthy Dinner Number 6

Pizza

Makes: 3 servings
Prep time: 8 minutes
Cook time: 10 minutes

Ingredients

Olive Oil
1 12-inch 100% whole wheat pizza crust
1 cup prepared tomato salsa
1/4 cup shredded reduced-fat 2% mozzarella
1 1/3 cups canned black beans, drained and rinsed
1 small sweet red pepper, seeded and thinly sliced (about 2/3 cup)
2 scallions, trimmed and thinly sliced
1/4 cup coriander leaves for garnish (optional)

Directions:

1. Heat the oven to 220° C. Place crust on sheet and top with salsa, mozzarella, beans, sliced red pepper, and scallions.

2. Place pizza in oven and bake 8 to 10 minutes or until mozzarella is melted. Remove from oven and garnish with coriander if desired. Cut into six slices and serve.

Healthy Dinner Number 7

Grilled Beef with Basil Puree over Tuscan Beans

Makes: 4 servings
Prep time: 10 minutes
Cook time: 10 minutes

Ingredients

1 teaspoon fresh lemon juice
1/4 cup extra virgin olive oil

1 ½ cups loosely packed fresh basil leaves
3 garlic cloves
1 teaspoon salt
1 teaspoon freshly ground black pepper
1 lb 1½ -inch-thick sirloin steak, cut into 4 portions
2 440g cans white beans, rinsed and drained
1 cup cherry tomatoes, halved
1 tablespoon finely chopped red onion

Directions:

1. In a food processor, combine the lemon juice, olive oil, 1 cup of the basil leaves, 1 garlic clove, 1/2 teaspoon of the salt, and 1/4 teaspoon of the black pepper. Puree until smooth; set aside.

2. Heat a grill to medium high. Halve one garlic clove and rub the steaks with its cut sides. Season meat with 1/4 teaspoon each of the salt and black pepper. Grill 5 to 6 minutes a side.

3. Mince remaining garlic and sauté in pan over medium-low heat for 2 minutes; let cool slightly. In a medium bowl, combine the white beans, tomatoes, red onion, remaining salt and black pepper, and sautéed garlic. Tear up remaining basil and combine with bean mixture.

4. Divide beans among four plates and top with steak. Add basil puree and serve.

Healthy Dinner Number 8

Chicken BLT Salad with Buttermilk Dressing

Makes: 4 servings
Prep time: 10 minutes
Cook time: 10 minutes

Ingredients

4 slices lean bacon (organic)
4 1-inch-thick slices ciabatta bread
2 teaspoons olive oil
1 garlic clove, halved
1/4 tablespoon light mayonnaise
2 teaspoons cider vinegar
1/4 teaspoon Dijon mustard
1/4 teaspoon minced garlic
1/4 teaspoon salt
1/8 teaspoon freshly ground black pepper
4 cups tightly packed chopped romaine lettuce
1 pint cherry tomatoes, halved
2 cups roughly torn chicken breast, skin removed

Directions:

1. Cook the bacon in a skillet over medium-low heat, turning occasionally, until lightly browned and beginning to crisp, about 6 minutes. Transfer to a paper-towel-lined plate to drain. Crumble into large pieces.

2. Heat a grill pan over medium-high heat. Lightly brush the ciabatta slices with the olive oil and grill until just toasted, about 2 minutes per side. Lightly rub the cut garlic clove halves over the surface of each slice. Let the bread cool then cut into 1-inch cubes.

3. In a large bowl, whisk together the buttermilk, mayonnaise, vinegar, mustard, minced garlic, salt, sugar, and black pepper. Add the lettuce, tomatoes, chicken, croutons, and half the bacon. Toss well. Transfer to plates and top each serving with some of the remaining bacon.

Healthy Dinner Number 9

Vegetable Curry

Makes: 6 servings
Prep time: 5 minutes, plus 5 extra minutes while the onion is cooking
Cook time: 15 minutes

Ingredients

1 tablespoon olive oil
1 large red onion, halved and cut into thin wedges
2 teaspoons curry powder
1 teaspoon ground cumin
1/4 teaspoon garam masala powder
1/8 teaspoon cayenne pepper
3 cups cauliflower florets
1 400g can diced tomatoes with liquid
2 medium potatoes, peeled and cut into 1-inch cubes (about 1 ½ cups)
2 medium sweet potatoes, peeled and cut into 1-inch cubes (about 1 ½ cups)
1 ½ cups vegetable stock or water
1/4 teaspoon salt
1/4 teaspoon black pepper
1 cup loose-pack frozen peas
4 ½ cups cooked couscous or brown rice

Directions:

1. Heat the olive oil in a large saucepan over medium heat. Add the onion and cook until tender, about 4 to 5 minutes. Add the curry powder, cumin, garam masala powder, and cayenne pepper. Stir well and cook for one minute.

2. Stir in the cauliflower, tomatoes, potatoes, sweet potatoes, stock, salt, and black pepper. Bring to the boil; reduce heat and simmer, covered, for 10 minutes or until the potatoes are tender. Stir in the peas; heat through. Serve over couscous or brown rice.

Healthy Dinner Number 10

Ancho-Glazed Salmon & Sweet Potato Fries

Makes: 4 servings
Start to finish: 20 minutes

Ingredients

> 1/4 tablespoon sugar
> 1 teaspoon salt
> 1 teaspoon ground cumin
> 1 teaspoon ground ancho chilli pepper or chilli powder
> 2 medium sweet potatoes, scrubbed
> Olive oil
> 4 skinless salmon fillets (5-6 ounces each)
> 1 tablespoon olive oil
> 2 tablespoons fresh coriander sprigs

Directions:

1. Preheat grill. In a small bowl, combine sugar, salt, cumin, and chilli powder. Cut sweet potatoes into 1/4-inch-thick slices. Coat sweet potatoes with olive oil and sprinkle with half the spice mixture. Grill 10 minutes, turning once halfway though.

2. Rinse and dry salmon; coat with remaining spice mixture. In a large skillet, cook fish in hot olive oil over medium heat for 4 minutes per side, or until it flakes easily with a fork.

3. Sprinkle sweet potatoes and salmon with coriander before serving.

Mindful Change

Over the next few days, I want you to work through the following exercises and immerse yourself into the patterns of changing your thinking. These exercises have been designed to help you change to new and supportive patterns.

You can do one per day, one every other day or even spread them out over the coming weeks – it doesn't matter. All that's important is that you accept you are accountable for your actions and that the commitment you make right now will generate your change in the future.

Mindful Change Exercise Number 1

TASK

Answer the following:

Why is weight loss important to me?

....

....

Having covered this in detail, we know that change will become easier after a period of time. To help keep you on track, I'd like you to write down the following rules. These should be placed prominently in the locations you are most likely to frequent on a daily basis.

Action 1 – I should only eat when I'm in a happy state of mind. If

I'm not happy then I should change my state before consuming food. If in doubt, drown it out (drink a glass of water with ice).

Action 2 – I will chew my food consciously, this will ensure that the messages reach my stomach and allow time for the mind to let me know I'm full.

Action 3 – I will give myself plenty of time to eat and prepare food; if I don't have the time then I will remove social media and TV from my life until I have the time.

Action 4 – I will always make myself consciously aware of what I am eating. Unless I know exactly what is in it, I won't be eating it. Who knows, it could be poison!

Action 5 – I will keep an honest and up to date diary of the food I am consuming, this includes everything that passes my lips – good, bad and neutral.

Although they seem overly simplistic and you may feel little need to write them down, the constant conscious reminder helps to improve your awareness of what you are doing and acts to change negative habits through re-patterning normal behaviours.

Mindful Change Exercise Number 2

TASK

Answer the following:

What do I want my body to look like and why?

....

....

We have already established that weight loss should not be the primary goal but rather the achievement of a healthy and supportive body.

Action 1 – Everything I eat is seen as energy and should be supportive to my mind and body: what can I do today to ensure that I only choose quality foods?

Action 2 – What can I do today to ensure that my body receives the right amount of movement required to tone and increase my cardiovascular performance?

Action 3 – What changes can I make today to the way I look to improve my own self-confidence?

Action 4 – Why do I deserve to be happy, loved and fulfilled in my life?

It's a fact that the more you work on you, the better you will be. Avoid the temptation to see yourself as a finished project; you have a number of years left to continue improving and live a better and more fulfilling life than you have already.

Mindful Change Exercise Number 3

TASK

Answer the following:

What conscious adjustments to food should I be making?

....

....

We know what we *should* be eating yet time and time again we kid ourselves that what we are actually eating won't matter – WRONG. Everything you consume – from a leftover chicken-dipper off your child's plate to a bottle of cola gulped down for a quick energy fix – matters.

Action 1 – Today I will be making a conscious choice to eat only 'real' foods rather than processed or 'fake' foods.

Action 2 – What can I remove from my usual working day that will remove all temptation to snack or consume food that has no positive nutritional value?

Action 3 – What new beliefs can I have about my body; why is now the right time to make the changes needed to improve my life for the better?

Action 4 – What can I do to reduce stress within my life today and begin moving forward with my life?

Conscious awareness of the foods we consume is essential to ensure that we continually make adjustments. Just as a ship requires adjustments to the sail, we also require the same level of conscious commitment to staying on course.

Mindful Change Exercise Number 4

TASK

Answer the following:

What can I do to ensure that I am eating the right amount of food?

....

....

Eating the right amount of food is essential in terms of overall health. Consuming too much will lead to your body storing the excess as fat but eating too little will slow your metabolism.

Action 1 – According to the RMR, what should I be eating per day to support my metabolism and the gradual reduction of body fat?

Action 2 – What can I do today to ensure that I'm not consuming food at the wrong time of the day?

Action 3 – How does planning help me with the right food choices?

Action 4 – How am I able to manage the intake of healthy food when eating out or without food that I have prepared?

Action 5 – Why am I eating healthy and nutritionally rich food?

Thinking in terms of 'actions' alters the way we communicate with ourselves, and by asking better questions we achieve better answers and better outcomes as a result.

Mindful Change Exercise Number 5

TASK

Answer the following:

Why am I so committed to change right now?

....

....

What am I going to do to ensure that I never relapse?

....

....

The Weight Loss Coach
How will I respond to people who look at my actions in a negative light?

....

....

Avoid the temptation to do more than you can, it will very rarely attract the results you want. This programme is not like other programmes, you are not restricted by time or goals, so take a moment to pause and think about what is realistically possible. If you have invested 20 years into achieving the weight you are now, accept that it's unrealistic to expect to lose unwanted weight in just a couple of weeks. Commit to getting on board for the journey and choose to make every change a lasting change.

The time is now and now is the time to begin discovering the best you it's possible to be.

But a word of warning: there are no quick fix solutions that support a long-term weight loss or lifestyle solution and there is no magic pill you can take over 12 weeks that will reverse the effects of poor lifestyle choices. Lasting change takes time; time to change your habits and time to adjust to new ways of being.

The best time to plant a tree was 20 years ago. The second best time is now.
–Chinese Proverb

Exercises

Walking Lunges:

1. Stand with your feet shoulder width apart and your hands on your hips.
2. Step forward with one leg, flexing (bending) the knees to drop your hips. Descend until your rear knee almost touches the ground. Your posture should remain upright, and your front knee should stay above the front foot.
3. Drive through the heel of your lead foot and extend (straighten) both knees to raise yourself back up.
4. Step forward with your rear foot, repeating the lunge on the opposite leg.

Lunges:

1. This exercise is best performed inside a squat rack for safety purposes. To begin, first set the bar on a rack just below shoulder level. Once the correct height is chosen and the bar is loaded, step under the bar and place the back of your shoulders (slightly below the neck) across it.
2. Hold on to the bar, placing one hand on each side of your shoulders, and lift it off the rack by first pushing with your legs and simultaneously straightening your torso.
3. Step away from the rack. Step forward with your right leg and squat down through your hips, while keeping the torso upright and maintaining balance. Inhale as you go down. Note: do not allow your knee to go forward beyond your toes as you come down as this will put undue stress on the knee joint.
4. Using mainly the heel of your foot, push up and go back to the starting position as you exhale.
5. Repeat the movement for the recommended amount of

repetitions and then perform with the left leg.

Squat:

1. Stand with your feet shoulder width apart. You can place your hands behind your head. This will be your starting position.
2. Begin the movement by flexing your knees and hips, sitting back with your hips as if about to sit down in an imaginary chair.
3. Continue down to full depth if you are able, and then quickly reverse the motion to return to the starting position. As you squat, keep your head and chest up and push your knees out.

Squat Jump:

1. Stand with your hands behind your head, and squat down keeping your torso upright and your head up. This will be your starting position.
2. Jump forward several feet, but avoid jumping unnecessarily high. As your feet contact the ground, absorb the impact through your legs, and jump again. Repeat this action 5-10 times.

Plank:

1. Get into a prone position (face down) on the floor, supporting your weight on your toes and your forearms. Your arms are bent with the elbows directly below the shoulders.
2. Keep your body straight – and hold. Maintain this position for as long as possible. To increase difficulty, an arm or leg can be raised from the floor.

Press Up:

1. Position yourself on your hands and knees on the floor. Adopt a press up (push up) position with your arms

perpendicular to the body, hips lower than shoulders (this can be achieved by positioning your hips further forwards than your knees) and body (back) straight.

2. Bend your elbows to lower your body towards the floor, inhale as you go, then push up by straightening your arms, exhaling as you return to the starting position.

Bent Over Row:

1. Place two dumbbells in front of your feet. Bend your knees slightly and push your butt out as much as possible. As you bend over to get into the starting position grab both dumbbells by the handles.
2. Pull one dumbbell off the floor while holding on to the other dumbbell. Retract the shoulder blade of the working side as you flex the elbow to draw the dumbbell towards your stomach or rib cage.
3. Lower the dumbbell and repeat the exercise with your other arm.

Shoulder Press:

1. Clean two dumbbells to your shoulders. Clean the dumbbells to your shoulders by extending through the legs and hips as you pull the dumbbells towards your shoulders. Rotate your wrists as you do so.
2. Press one dumbbell directly overhead by extending through the elbow, turning it so the palm faces forward while holding the other dumbbell in place by your shoulder.
3. Lower the pressed dumbbell to the starting position and immediately press with the other arm.

Upright Row:

1. Grab a dumbbell in each arm and stand up straight with your arms extended by your sides, keeping a slight bend in your elbows. This will be your starting position. Tip: the dumbbells should be next to your thighs with the palms of your hands facing backwards.

2. Use your shoulders to lift the dumbbells up and out from your body with elbows leading the movement. Aim to raise the dumbbells to a height that's in line with your chin, exhale as you lift. Tip: as you lift the dumbbells, your elbows should always be higher than your forearms. Keep your torso still (no rocking or swinging to assist the lift) and pause for a second at the top of the movement.
3. Lower the dumbbells slowly back down to the starting position. Inhale as you do so.
4. Repeat for the recommended amount of repetitions.

Bicep Curl:

1. Stand up straight with a dumbbell in each hand at arm's length – arms by your sides. Keeping your elbows close to your torso, rotate the palms of your hands until they are facing forward. This will be your starting position.
2. Keeping the upper arms fixed in place, curl the weights while contracting your biceps to raise your hands towards your shoulders. Exhale as you do so. Continue to raise the weights until your biceps are fully contracted and the dumbbells are at shoulder level. Hold the contracted position for a brief pause as you squeeze your biceps.
3. Slowly begin to lower the dumbbells back to the starting position, inhale as you go.
4. Repeat for the recommended amount of repetitions.

Triceps Extensions:

1. Grab a dumbbell and sit on a military press bench or a utility bench that has a back support on it. Place the dumbbell on top of your thigh.
2. Clean the dumbbell to bring it up to shoulder height and then extend the arm so that the weight is being held over your head with a straight arm. Use your other arm to support the raised arm if necessary (hold the upper arm in place).
3. Rotate the wrist on the raised arm so that the palm of your

hand is facing forward and bend your elbow slightly so that the pinkie is facing the ceiling. This will be your starting position.

4. Slowly lower the dumbbell behind your head by bending your elbow, keeping the upper arm in place by your head. Inhale as you perform this movement and pause when your triceps are fully stretched.

5. Return to the starting position by flexing your triceps, exhale as you raise the dumbbell. Tip: it is imperative that only the forearm moves. The upper arm should remain in position next to your head at all times.

6. Repeat for the recommended amount of repetitions and switch arms.

Crawl Out:

1. Begin in a prone position on the floor. Support your weight on your hands and toes, with your feet together and your body straight. Your arms should be bent to 90 degrees. This will be your starting position.

2. Crawl out five paces then return to the starting point.

Burpees

1. Stand with your feet hip width apart and your arms down by your side.

2. Lower into a squat position and place your hands flat on the floor in front of you.

3. Kick your legs out backwards into a press up position and lower your chest to the floor.

4. Push your chest back up to the press up position as you jump both feet forward to return to the squat position.

5. Jump up and raise both hands over your head.

Crunches:

1. Lie flat on your back with your feet flat on the ground, or resting on a bench with your knees bent at a 90 degree angle. If you are resting your feet on a bench, place them

three to four inches apart and point your toes inward so they touch.

2. Place your hands lightly on either side of your head keeping your elbows in. Tip: don't lock your fingers behind your head as this will lead to pulling on your neck..

3. While pushing the small of your back down into the floor to better isolate your abdominal muscles, begin to roll your shoulders off the floor.

4. Continue to push down as hard as you can with your lower back as you contract your abdominals and exhale. Your shoulders should come up off the floor only about four inches, and your lower back should remain on the floor. At the top of the movement, contract your abdominals tightly and keep the contraction for a second. Tip: focus on slow, controlled movement – don't cheat yourself by using momentum.

5. After the one second contraction, slowly return to the starting position as you inhale.

6. Repeat for the recommended amount of repetitions.

Oblique Crunch:

1. Start out by lying on your right side with your legs lying on top of each other. Make sure your knees are slightly bent.

2. Place your left hand behind your head.

3. Once you are in this starting position, begin to crunch by imagining your left elbow is aiming towards your left hip.

4. Crunch as high as you can, hold the contraction for a second and then slowly drop back down into the starting position.

5. Exhale as you crunch up, inhale as you return to the starting position.

Reverse Curl:

1. Stand up straight with hips placed shoulder-width apart. Hold a dumbbell in each hand, holding each one with an overhand grip so that your palms will face the floor as you

curl. This is the starting position.

2. Keeping the upper arms fixed in place, curl the weights while contracting the biceps to raise the back of your hands towards your shoulders. Exhale as you do so. Continue to raise the weights until your biceps are fully contracted and the dumbbells are at shoulder level. Hold the contracted position for a brief pause as you squeeze your biceps. Tip: only the forearms should move.

3. Slowly begin to lower the dumbbells back to starting position as your breathe in.

4. Repeat for the recommended amount of repetitions.

Cross Over Crunch:

1. Lie flat on your back and bend your knees about 60 degrees.

2. Keep your feet flat on the floor and place your hands loosely behind your head. This will be your starting position.

3. Curl up by crunching your abdominal muscles and bring your right elbow and shoulder across your body to meet your left knee as you raise your left foot from the floor. Reach with your elbow and try to touch your knee. Exhale as you perform this movement. Tip: try to bring your shoulder up towards your knee rather than just your elbow and remember that the key is to contract the abs as you perform the movement, not just move the elbow.

4. Return to the starting position as you inhale and repeat with the left elbow and right knee.

5. Continue alternating in this manner until all prescribed repetitions are done.

Bicycle crunches:

1. Lie flat on the floor with your lower back pressed to the ground. For this exercise, you will need to place your hands on your temples but be careful not to strain your neck by attempting to lift your head. Raise your shoulders off the floor into the crunch position.

2. Raise your feet off the floor and bend your legs into a 90 degree angle (thighs perpendicular and lower legs parallel to the floor). This will be your starting position.

3. Begin a cycle motion by bringing your left knee inwards to meet your right elbow while simultaneously straightening out your right leg away from your body.

4. Return to the start position then continue the cycle motion by this time bringing your right knee inwards to meet your left elbow while straightening out your left leg at the same time.

5. Continue alternating in this manner until all of the recommended repetitions for each side have been completed.

Kick Out:

1. Kneel on the floor or an exercise mat and bend at the waist with your arms extended in front of you (perpendicular to the torso) in order to get into a kneeling push-up position, but with your arms spaced at shoulder width. Your head should be looking forward and the bend of the knees should create a 90-degree angle between the hamstrings and the calves. This will be your starting position.

2. As you exhale, lift up your right leg until the hamstrings are in line with your back while maintaining the 90-degree angle in your knee. Contract the glutes (butt) throughout this movement and hold the contraction at the top for a second. Tip: at the end of the movement, the upper leg should be parallel to the floor while the calf should be perpendicular to it.

3. Return to the starting position as you inhale and then repeat with the left leg.

4. Continue to alternate legs until all of the recommended repetitions have been performed.

Squat Thrust:

1. Clean two kettlebells to your shoulders. Clean the

kettlebells to your shoulders by extending through the legs and hips as you pull the kettlebells towards your shoulders. Rotate your wrists as you do so. This will be your starting position.

2. Begin to squat by flexing your hips and knees, lowering your hips between your legs. Maintain an upright, straight back as you squat as low as you can.

3. At the bottom, reverse direction by extending your knees and hips, driving through your heels. As you do so, press both kettlebells overhead by extending your arms over head, using the momentum from the squat to help drive the weights upward.

4. As you begin the next repetition, return the weights to the shoulders.

About Benjamin Bonetti

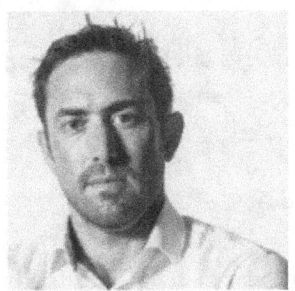

Benjamin Bonetti is considered one of the leading authorities within the self-help arena and has produced several leading hypnosis products.

Bonetti promotes and writes about the power of positive thinking and the essential need to take massive action. He is known to talk about his early struggles and refers to them in several of his early written pieces as the building blocks to his success.

Over the last 10 years his therapy techniques and bullish tactics have attracted many critics who believe that the no-nonsense approach can be interpreted as too forceful, especially to those with more sensitive issues. Bonetti, however, believes that it is this technique that is often overlooked by more "fluffy" type therapies and is the reason behind relapses.

Bonetti started his career in the British Army, serving for several years until later pursuing his dream of owning his own business; his entrepreneurial spirit has led him to own several businesses and later establish Benjamin Bonetti Ltd.

Bonetti has several well-known family links, and is related to Peter Bonetti (The Cat) the English goal keeper whose successful career saw him playing for both Chelsea and England during the 1970s.

Outside of business, Bonetti has been seen to promote the "voice" of the youth and during 2004 stood for local election, as the youngest person in history for that Council. Bonetti is also a keen and active conservationist, and volunteers for various countryside management organizations.

Although many of Bonetti's clients still remain unknown, he is often spotted behind the scenes at events supporting known A-list celebrities and artists. During a 2009 New Year's Day interview with the BBC Asian Network, Bonetti was referred to as a "celebrity must have secret weapon."

The success of his personal development audio recordings have led to them being available internationally, including in the UK, Ireland, Mexico, the USA, Australia, New Zealand, and Hong Kong.

http://www.benjaminbonetti.com
Facebook: Benjamin Bonetti

Also Available:

Books

- Fat Body Fat Mind: Createspace, 2012 – ISBN 1479167355
- Don't Struggle Quietly: Createspace, 2012 – ISBN 1475153422
- Inspirational & Motivational Quotes: Createspace, 2010 – ISBN 1456333658
- Entrepreneurs Always Drive On Empty: Createspace, 2010 – ISBN 1453771093

Seminars & Training:
- The Law Of Attraction – The Truth
- NLP Practitioner Training UK & Overseas
- NLP Master Practitioner Training UK & Overseas

Bonetti has produced a wide range of Hypnosis CDs and MP3s. The value of these is unknown to date, but consist of one of the largest ranges of hypnosis recordings by any one person.

- The Easy Way to Lose Weight with Hypnosis, Audiogo: 2013. ISBN 1471326284
- The Easy Way to Beat Insomnia and Sleep Easy with Hypnosis, Audiogo: 2013. ISBN 1471326322
- The Easy Way to Increase Self Confidence with Hyp- nosis, Audiogo: 2013. ISBN 1471326306
- The Easy Way to Stop Smoking with Hypnosis, Audiogo: 2013. ISBN 1471326314
- The Easy Way to Become Stress Free with Hypnosis, Audiogo: 2013. ISBN 1471326292

2013 Advance Hypnotic Technique Audios MP3s
- The Easy Way to Lose Weight with Hypnosis, Audiogo: 2013. ASIN: B00ANZ392S
- The Easy Way to Increase Self-Confidence with Hyp- nosis,

Audiogo: 2013. ASIN: B00ANZ32ZW

• The Easy Way to Stop Smoking with Hypnosis, Audiogo: 2013. ASIN: B00ANZ37DO

• The Easy Way to Beat Insomnia and Sleep Easy with Hypnosis, Audiogo: 2013. ASIN: B00ANZ38CY

• The Easy and Original Hypnotic Gastric Band, Audiogo: 2013. ASIN: B00ANZ36OY

• The Easy Way to Relax during Pregnancy, Audiogo: 2013. ASIN: B00ANZ30R2

• The Easy Way to Beat Nail Biting with Hypnosis, Audiogo: 2013. ASIN: B00ANZ31K8

• The Easy Way to Improve Self-Belief with Hypnosis, Audiogo: 2013. ASIN: B00ANZ326G

• The Easy Way to Overcome Anxiety with Hypnosis, Audiogo: 2013. ASIN: B00ANZ35EU

• The Easy Way to Become Stress Free with Hypnosis, Audiogo: 2013. ASIN: B00ANZ3036